ATKINS DIET COOKBOOK FOR SENIORS

The ultimate guide to Delicious Low-Carb recipes to boost energy, improve health and enjoy life

DR. Jeanette Reeves

All rights reserved. No part of this publication may be reproduced, distributed, or transmitted in any form or by any means, including photocopying, recording, or other electronic or mechanical methods, without the prior written permission of the publisher, except in the case of brief quotations embodied in critical reviews and certain other noncommercial uses permitted by copyright law.

Copyright © DR.Jeanette Reeves, 2024.

Table of contents

Chapter 1. Introduction to Atkins Diet for Seniors

- Understanding the Atkins Diet

As we age, our dietary needs change, and prioritizing health becomes increasingly important. The Atkins Diet offers seniors a unique approach to nutrition, focusing on low-carbohydrate, high-protein meals to promote weight loss, improve energy levels, and support overall wellness.

In this introductory section, we will delve into the fundamentals of the Atkins Diet and explore its potential benefits for seniors. We'll discuss how this dietary approach can help address common health concerns associated with aging, such as weight management, blood sugar regulation, and cardiovascular health.

By understanding the principles of the Atkins Diet and learning how to adapt it to suit the needs of seniors, you can embark on a journey towards better health and vitality in your golden years. Whether you're looking to shed excess pounds, boost your energy levels, or simply adopt a healthier lifestyle, the Atkins Diet offers a flexible and effective solution that can be tailored to fit your individual needs and preferences. Let's explore the transformative power of the Atkins Diet and discover how it can help you achieve your health goals as a senior.

Understanding the Atkins Diet as a senior involves recognizing its core principles and how they can be tailored to meet the unique nutritional needs and health concerns of older adults. Here's a breakdown of key points to consider:

1. Low-Carb Approach: The Atkins Diet emphasizes reducing carbohydrate intake to control blood sugar levels and promote weight loss. As a senior, this can be particularly beneficial for managing conditions like diabetes or prediabetes, which become more common with age.

2. Focus on Protein and Healthy Fats: Seniors need adequate protein to support muscle maintenance and repair, as well as healthy fats for brain function and hormone production. The Atkins Diet encourages the consumption of protein-rich foods like lean meats, fish, eggs, and tofu, along with sources of healthy fats such as avocados, nuts, seeds, and olive oil.

3. Weight Management: Many seniors struggle with maintaining a healthy weight due to factors like reduced muscle mass and slower metabolism. The Atkins Diet can help address this by promoting fat loss while preserving muscle mass, which is essential for maintaining mobility and overall health in later years.

4. Blood Sugar Regulation: Seniors are at higher risk for insulin resistance and type 2 diabetes, making blood sugar management a priority. By minimizing carbohydrate intake and focusing on low-glycemic foods, the Atkins Diet can help stabilize blood sugar levels and reduce the risk of diabetes-related complications.

5. Bone Health Adequate protein intake is crucial for maintaining bone density and preventing osteoporosis, a common concern for seniors. The Atkins Diet encourages the consumption of protein-rich foods that also provide essential nutrients like calcium and vitamin D, which are important for bone health.

6. Heart Health: Seniors are more susceptible to heart disease, so it's important to follow a heart-healthy diet. While the Atkins Diet initially garnered criticism for its high-fat content, newer versions emphasize healthy fats from sources like nuts, seeds, and fatty fish, which can have a positive impact on heart health when consumed in moderation.

7. Digestive Health: Many seniors experience digestive issues such as constipation or gastrointestinal discomfort. The Atkins Diet promotes the consumption of fiber-rich vegetables and low-carb fruits, which can support digestive health and regularity.

 - Benefits of the Atkins Diet for Seniors

The Atkins Diet offers several potential benefits for seniors, catering to their unique nutritional needs and health concerns. Here are some key advantages of the Atkins Diet for older adults:

1. Weight Management: As metabolism tends to slow down with age, many seniors struggle with weight gain or find it challenging to lose excess pounds. The Atkins Diet's low-carb approach

can be effective for weight management, promoting fat loss while preserving muscle mass. This can lead to improved body composition and a healthier weight, reducing the risk of obesity-related health issues such as heart disease, diabetes, and joint problems.

2. Blood Sugar Control: Seniors are at higher risk for insulin resistance and type 2 diabetes, making blood sugar management a priority. By minimizing carbohydrate intake and focusing on low-glycemic foods, the Atkins Diet can help stabilize blood sugar levels and reduce the risk of diabetes-related complications. This can improve overall health and quality of life for seniors with diabetes or prediabetes.

3. Cardiovascular Health: While earlier versions of the Atkins Diet were criticized for their high saturated fat content, newer iterations emphasize healthy fats from sources like nuts, seeds, and fatty fish. These fats have been shown to have a positive impact on heart health, reducing the risk of heart disease and stroke. By incorporating heart-healthy fats and limiting refined carbohydrates, the Atkins Diet can support cardiovascular health in seniors.

4. Muscle Preservation: Maintaining muscle mass is crucial for seniors to support mobility, independence, and overall quality of life. The protein-rich nature of the Atkins Diet helps preserve muscle mass while promoting fat loss, which can be particularly beneficial for older adults who may be at risk of sarcopenia or age-related muscle loss. Adequate protein intake also supports muscle repair and recovery, especially for seniors who engage in physical activity or strength training.

5. Brain Health: Healthy fats, such as those found in avocados, olive oil, and fatty fish, are essential for brain function and cognitive health. The Atkins Diet encourages the consumption of these nutrient-dense fats, which can support cognitive function and reduce the risk of age-related cognitive decline and neurodegenerative diseases like Alzheimer's.

6. Stable Energy Levels: Many seniors experience fluctuations in energy levels throughout the day, which can impact daily activities and quality of life. By reducing reliance on carbohydrates

for energy and focusing on protein and healthy fats, the Atkins Diet can provide a more stable source of energy, helping seniors feel more alert, focused, and energized throughout the day.

7. Digestive Health: The Atkins Diet emphasizes whole, nutrient-dense foods like vegetables, nuts, and seeds, which are rich in fiber and promote digestive health. For seniors who may experience digestive issues like constipation or gastrointestinal discomfort, a diet high in fiber can help alleviate symptoms and support regularity.

8. Joint Health: Excess weight can put strain on the joints, leading to pain and discomfort, especially in seniors with conditions like osteoarthritis. By promoting weight loss and reducing inflammation through its low-carb, nutrient-dense approach, the Atkins Diet can help alleviate joint pain and improve mobility, allowing seniors to stay active and engaged in daily activities.

9. Reduced Risk of Chronic Diseases: The Atkins Diet's focus on whole, unprocessed foods and its emphasis on reducing refined carbohydrates can help lower the risk of chronic diseases commonly associated with aging, such as heart disease, stroke, and certain types of cancer. By supporting overall health and well-being, the Atkins Diet can help seniors enjoy a higher quality of life as they age.

10. Improved Sleep Quality: Sleep disturbances are common among seniors and can have a significant impact on overall health and well-being. Research suggests that dietary factors, including carbohydrate intake, can affect sleep quality. By stabilizing blood sugar levels and promoting a more balanced intake of nutrients, the Atkins Diet may help improve sleep patterns and promote better rest for seniors.

11. Mental Well-being: Proper nutrition plays a vital role in mental health and well-being, especially as we age. The Atkins Diet encourages the consumption of nutrient-rich foods like fruits, vegetables, and lean proteins, which provide essential vitamins, minerals, and antioxidants that support brain health and mood regulation. By nourishing the body and brain with healthy fats and proteins, the Atkins Diet can contribute to improved mental clarity, focus, and overall cognitive function in seniors.

12. Increased Longevity: By supporting overall health and reducing the risk of chronic diseases, the Atkins Diet may contribute to increased longevity and a higher quality of life in older adults. By adopting healthy eating habits and lifestyle changes, seniors can enjoy more active, fulfilling years well into their golden years.

Overall, the Atkins Diet offers seniors a flexible and effective approach to nutrition that can help address common health concerns associated with aging, promote weight management, stabilize blood sugar levels, support cardiovascular and brain health, preserve muscle mass, and improve overall well-being and quality of life.

- How the Atkins Diet can Support Senior Health

The Atkins Diet offers multifaceted support for senior health by addressing key nutritional needs and health concerns commonly associated with aging. By emphasizing a low-carbohydrate, high-protein approach, the Atkins Diet helps seniors manage weight more effectively, reducing the risk of obesity-related conditions such as heart disease, diabetes, and joint problems. Additionally, the diet's focus on protein-rich foods supports muscle maintenance and repair, essential for preserving mobility, strength, and independence as seniors age. Stable blood sugar levels are crucial for managing diabetes and preventing related complications, and the Atkins Diet's carbohydrate restriction helps stabilize glucose levels, supporting better overall health and quality of life for seniors with diabetes or prediabetes. Furthermore, by prioritizing healthy fats from sources like nuts, seeds, and fatty fish, the Atkins Diet promotes heart health and cognitive function, reducing the risk of cardiovascular disease and age-related cognitive decline. Improved energy levels, better sleep quality, and enhanced mental well-being are additional benefits seniors may experience on the Atkins Diet, contributing to a more active, fulfilling lifestyle in their later years. Overall, the Atkins Diet offers seniors a comprehensive approach to nutrition and health, empowering them to age gracefully and enjoy optimal well-being well into their golden years.

<u>**Chapter 2. Getting Started with the Atkins Diet**</u>

- Preparing for the Atkins Diet

Preparing for the Atkins Diet as a woman over 60 involves several key steps to ensure success and safety:

1. Understand the phases: The Atkins Diet consists of four phases – Induction, Ongoing Weight Loss, Pre-Maintenance, and Maintenance. Each phase has specific guidelines regarding carbohydrate intake. Understanding these phases and how they progress will help you navigate the diet effectively.

2. Plan your meals: Take time to plan your meals in advance, focusing on whole foods such as lean proteins, healthy fats, and low-carb vegetables. Incorporate a variety of foods to ensure you're getting a balance of nutrients.

3. Stock up on low-carb foods: Fill your kitchen with Atkins-friendly foods like meats, fish, eggs, cheese, nuts, seeds, and low-carb vegetables. Having these options readily available will make it easier to stick to the diet and avoid temptation.

4. Stay hydrated: Drink plenty of water throughout the day to stay hydrated and support your body's functions. Aim for at least eight glasses of water per day, or more if you're exercising or in a hot climate.

5. Monitor your progress: Keep track of your food intake, carbohydrate consumption, and any changes in weight or measurements. This will help you gauge your progress and make adjustments as needed.

6. Be mindful of portion sizes: While the Atkins Diet doesn't restrict calories, it's still important to be mindful of portion sizes to avoid overeating. Pay attention to hunger cues and stop eating when you feel satisfied

7. Incorporate physical activity: Regular exercise is an important component of a healthy lifestyle, especially when following a diet plan. Aim for a combination of cardiovascular exercise, strength training, and flexibility exercises to support your overall health and well-being.

8. Listen to your body: Pay attention to how your body responds to the Atkins Diet. If you experience any adverse effects or discomfort, such as fatigue, constipation, or dizziness, adjust your diet accordingly.

9. Seek support: Consider joining a support group or finding a diet buddy to share your experiences, challenges, and successes with. Having a support system can provide motivation and encouragement along your journey.

10. Focus on nutrient density: As you age, it becomes even more important to prioritize nutrient-dense foods to support overall health and vitality. Choose foods rich in vitamins, minerals, and antioxidants, such as leafy greens, colorful vegetables, berries, and healthy fats like avocado and olive oil.

11. Be mindful of bone health: Women over 60 are at a higher risk of osteoporosis and bone fractures. Ensure you're getting an adequate intake of calcium and vitamin D through sources like dairy products, leafy greens, fortified foods, and supplements if necessary.

12. Consider potential medication interactions: If you're taking any medications, be aware that the Atkins Diet may interact with certain medications, particularly those for diabetes, high blood pressure, or cholesterol. Consult with your healthcare provider to ensure your medication regimen is compatible with the diet plan.

13. Adapt the diet to your individual needs: While the Atkins Diet provides general guidelines, it's important to tailor the plan to suit your unique preferences, dietary restrictions, and lifestyle. Experiment with different recipes, meal timings, and food combinations to find what works best for you.

14. Manage potential side effects: Some people may experience side effects when first starting the Atkins Diet, such as the "keto flu" (fatigue, headaches, irritability) during the induction phase. These symptoms are usually temporary and can be alleviated by staying hydrated, consuming electrolytes, and gradually increasing your carbohydrate intake.

15. Prioritize sleep and stress management: Adequate sleep and stress management are crucial for overall health and weight management, especially as we age. Aim for 7-9 hours of quality sleep per night and incorporate stress-reducing activities such as meditation, yoga, or gentle exercise into your daily routine.

16. Be patient and realistic: Weight loss may occur more slowly as you age, so it's important to be patient and realistic with your expectations. Focus on the health benefits of the diet beyond just weight loss, such as improved energy levels, blood sugar control, and cognitive function.

17. Monitor other health markers: In addition to tracking your weight and measurements, consider monitoring other health markers such as blood pressure, blood sugar levels, cholesterol levels, and inflammation markers. This comprehensive approach will give you a more holistic view of your health and progress.

18. Hormonal changes: Women over 60 may experience hormonal changes such as menopause or fluctuations in estrogen levels. These changes can impact metabolism, appetite, and body composition. Be mindful of how these factors may influence your experience with the Atkins Diet and adjust your approach accordingly.

19. Muscle mass preservation: As we age, maintaining muscle mass becomes increasingly important for overall health and functional independence. Ensure you're consuming adequate protein on the Atkins Diet to support muscle maintenance and repair. Aim for a variety of protein sources, including lean meats, poultry, fish, eggs, and plant-based options like tofu and legumes.

20. Gut health: The Atkins Diet may affect gut health due to changes in dietary fiber intake and the types of foods consumed. To support a healthy gut microbiome, include fiber-rich vegetables,

nuts, seeds, and low-sugar fruits in your diet. Fermented foods like yogurt, kefir, sauerkraut, and kimchi can also promote digestive health.

21. Psychological well-being: Dieting, especially in older age, can have psychological implications such as stress, anxiety, or feelings of deprivation. Practice self-care strategies to nurture your mental and emotional well-being, such as mindfulness, relaxation techniques, hobbies, social activities, and seeking support from friends and family.

22. Social dynamics: Social gatherings and cultural norms around food may present challenges when following a low-carb diet like Atkins. Communicate your dietary preferences and goals to friends, family, and hosts, and be proactive in finding low-carb options or bringing your own dishes to events.

23. Long-term sustainability: Consider the long-term sustainability of the Atkins Diet and how it fits into your lifestyle and preferences. While the initial phases may involve strict carbohydrate restriction, the Maintenance phase allows for more flexibility and gradual reintroduction of carbs. Focus on developing healthy eating habits that you can maintain for the long term, rather than viewing the diet as a short-term fix.

By following these tips and taking a proactive approach to your health, you can set yourself up for success on the Atkins Diet as a woman over 60.

- Setting Realistic Goals

Setting realistic goals is crucial for success when starting the Atkins Diet as a woman over 60. Here's a guide to help you set achievable and meaningful goals:

1. Understand your motivations: Reflect on why you're starting the Atkins Diet and what you hope to achieve. Whether it's weight loss, improved energy levels, better blood sugar control, or overall health and well-being, understanding your motivations will help you set goals that are meaningful to you.

2. Be specific and measurable: Instead of setting vague goals like "lose weight" or "eat healthier," make your goals specific and measurable. For example, aim to lose a certain number of pounds within a specified time frame or to reduce your intake of refined carbs by a certain percentage.

3. Break goals into smaller milestones: Break larger goals into smaller, more manageable milestones. This can help prevent overwhelm and allow you to celebrate progress along the way. For example, if your ultimate goal is to lose 20 pounds, set smaller milestones of 5 pounds each.

4. Set realistic timelines: Be realistic about the time it will take to achieve your goals. Rapid weight loss may not be sustainable or healthy, especially for older adults. Aim for gradual, sustainable progress, and be patient with yourself.

5. Consider non-scale victories: While weight loss may be a primary goal, consider other markers of success such as improved energy levels, better sleep, increased physical fitness, or reductions in medications (with guidance from your healthcare provider).

6. Focus on health outcomes: Shift your focus from just the number on the scale to overall health outcomes. Measure success by improvements in blood sugar levels, cholesterol levels, blood pressure, mobility, or quality of life.

7. Be flexible and adaptable: Life happens, and setbacks are a natural part of any journey. Be prepared to adjust your goals and strategies as needed, and don't be too hard on yourself if you encounter obstacles along the way.

8. Track your progress: Keep track of your food intake, physical activity, and any changes in weight or measurements. This will allow you to monitor your progress and make adjustments as necessary. Consider keeping a food journal or using a tracking app to stay accountable.

9. Celebrate achievements: Celebrate your successes, no matter how small. Acknowledge your hard work and dedication, and reward yourself in non-food ways that align with your goals and values.

10. Consider lifestyle factors: Take into account your current lifestyle, responsibilities, and commitments when setting goals. Consider how the Atkins Diet can fit into your daily routine and what adjustments you may need to make to support your goals effectively.

11. Focus on behavior changes: Instead of solely focusing on outcomes like weight loss, prioritize behavior changes that support long-term success. This might include adopting healthier eating habits, incorporating regular physical activity, practicing mindful eating, or managing stress more effectively.

12. Set process-oriented goals: Instead of fixating on the end result, focus on the actions and behaviors that will lead you there. For example, set goals related to meal planning, cooking nutritious meals at home, trying new low-carb recipes, or increasing your daily activity level.

13. Be realistic about challenges: Anticipate potential challenges or obstacles that may arise along the way, such as social events, holidays, travel, or cravings for high-carb foods. Develop strategies for how you'll navigate these challenges while staying committed to your goals.

14. Seek support: Surround yourself with a supportive network of friends, family members, or fellow Atkins dieters who can encourage and motivate you throughout your journey. Consider joining online forums, support groups, or local meetups to connect with others who are on a similar path.

15. Practice self-compassion: Be kind to yourself and practice self-compassion, especially if you experience setbacks or difficulties. Remember that progress is not always linear, and it's okay to have moments of struggle. Treat yourself with the same kindness and understanding that you would offer to a friend in a similar situation.

16. Reassess and readjust as needed: Periodically reassess your goals and progress to determine if any adjustments are necessary. If you find that certain goals are no longer realistic or relevant, don't hesitate to modify them accordingly. Flexibility and adaptability are key to long-term success.

17. Focus on overall well-being: Remember that health is about more than just the number on the scale. Prioritize your overall well-being, including physical, mental, and emotional health, as you pursue your goals on the Atkins Diet.

   - Overcoming Challenges as a woman over 60

Starting any new diet, including the Atkins Diet, can present challenges, especially for women over 60. Here are some strategies to help you overcome common challenges and stay on track:

1. Gradual Transition: Instead of diving headfirst into the Atkins Diet, consider gradually reducing your carbohydrate intake over a period of time. This can help minimize potential side effects like the "keto flu" and make the transition more manageable.

2. Meal Planning: Plan your meals and snacks in advance to ensure you have plenty of Atkins-friendly options on hand. Stock your kitchen with low-carb foods like lean proteins, vegetables, healthy fats, and sugar-free snacks to make meal prep easier.

3. Cravings: Cravings for high-carb foods can be a challenge, especially in the beginning stages of the Atkins Diet. Combat cravings by incorporating satisfying, low-carb alternatives into your diet, such as nuts, seeds, cheese, and sugar-free desserts.

4. Social Situations: Social gatherings, dinners out, and family events can be tricky to navigate on a low-carb diet. Plan ahead by checking menus in advance, bringing a dish to share that fits your dietary needs, or eating a small, satisfying meal before the event to avoid temptation.

5. Plateaus: It's common to experience weight loss plateaus or stalls, especially as your body adjusts to a new way of eating. If you hit a plateau, don't get discouraged. Focus on non-scale victories like improved energy levels, better sleep, or reductions in body measurements.

6. Physical Activity: Incorporating regular physical activity into your routine can support weight loss and overall health on the Atkins Diet. Choose activities that you enjoy and that are appropriate for your fitness level, whether it's walking, swimming, yoga, or strength training.

7. Medical Considerations: Women over 60 may have specific medical considerations that need to be taken into account when starting a new diet. Before beginning the Atkins Diet, ensure it's safe and appropriate for you, especially if you have any underlying health conditions or take medications.

8. Hydration: Adequate hydration is important on the Atkins Diet, especially during the initial phases when your body is adjusting to lower carbohydrate intake. Drink plenty of water throughout the day and consider incorporating herbal teas or flavored sparkling water for variety.

9. Mindset: Adopting a positive mindset and staying motivated are key to overcoming challenges on the Atkins Diet. Remind yourself of your reasons for starting the diet, set realistic goals, and celebrate your successes along the way.

10. Seek Support: Don't be afraid to reach out for support from friends, family members, or online communities of fellow Atkins dieters. Sharing your experiences, struggles, and successes with others who understand can provide encouragement and motivation.

11. Manage Digestive Changes: As we age, digestive issues such as constipation or gastrointestinal discomfort may become more common. Ensure you're getting enough fiber from low-carb vegetables, nuts, seeds, and other sources, and stay hydrated to support healthy digestion. If needed, consider incorporating natural remedies or supplements recommended by your healthcare provider.

12. Mindful Eating: Practice mindful eating to enhance your awareness of hunger and fullness cues, as well as the sensory experience of eating. Slow down, savor each bite, and pay attention to how different foods make you feel physically and emotionally. This can help prevent overeating and promote satisfaction with your meals.

13. Address Emotional Eating: Emotional eating, or turning to food for comfort or stress relief, can derail your efforts on the Atkins Diet. Develop alternative coping strategies for managing emotions, such as journaling, meditation, deep breathing exercises, or engaging in hobbies and activities you enjoy.

14. Adjust for Hormonal Changes: Hormonal changes associated with menopause or aging can affect appetite, metabolism, and weight management. Be patient and understanding with your body as it adapts to these changes, and consider strategies to support hormone balance, such as stress reduction techniques, adequate sleep, and regular physical activity.

15. Monitor Blood Sugar Levels: If you have diabetes or insulin resistance, closely monitor your blood sugar levels as you adjust to the Atkins Diet. Make sure your medications are properly adjusted and that you're managing your blood sugar effectively through diet, exercise, and medication as needed.

16. Focus on Whole Foods: Prioritize whole, minimally processed foods on the Atkins Diet to maximize nutrient intake and support overall health. Choose nutrient-dense options like lean proteins, healthy fats, and colorful vegetables, and limit highly processed or artificial foods that may be low in carbs but lacking in nutritional value.

17. Practice Self-Care: Make self-care a priority as you embark on your Atkins Diet journey. Set aside time for activities that nourish your mind, body, and soul, such as gentle exercise, relaxation techniques, spending time in nature, or indulging in hobbies and interests that bring you joy.

18. Celebrate Progress: Celebrate your achievements and milestones along the way, no matter how small. Recognize the effort and dedication you're putting into improving your health and well-being, and acknowledge the positive changes you're making in your life.

19. Stay Flexible: Be flexible and adaptable in your approach to the Atkins Diet, especially as you navigate potential challenges or setbacks. Remember that it's okay to modify your goals or strategies as needed to better suit your individual needs and circumstances.

20. Stay Positive: Maintain a positive attitude and mindset throughout your Atkins Diet journey. Focus on the progress you've made and the positive changes you're experiencing, and use any challenges or setbacks as opportunities for growth and learning.

- Kitchen Essentials for women

Here's a list of kitchen essentials that a woman over 60 starting the Atkins diet should consider having:

1. Food Scale: A food scale can help you accurately measure portions of protein, vegetables, and other foods to ensure you're staying within your carb limits.

2. Measuring Cups and Spoons: These are essential for measuring ingredients like nuts, seeds, oils, and sauces to maintain portion control and accuracy in your meal preparation.

3. Quality Knives: Invest in a set of sharp, high-quality knives for chopping, slicing, and dicing vegetables, meats, and other ingredients with ease.

4. Cutting Board: A sturdy cutting board is essential for food preparation and helps protect your countertops and knives.

5. Cookware Set: A basic set of pots and pans, including a skillet, saucepan, and stockpot, will cover most of your cooking needs. Opt for non-stick or stainless steel options.

6. Baking Sheet: Use a baking sheet for roasting vegetables, baking low-carb treats, or cooking proteins like chicken breasts or fish fillets.

7. Blender or Food Processor: A blender or food processor is handy for making smoothies, sauces, soups, and homemade dressings.

8. Vegetable Spiralizer: This tool allows you to turn vegetables like zucchini, squash, or carrots into low-carb "noodles" for pasta alternatives.

9. Salad Spinner: A salad spinner makes it easy to wash and dry leafy greens and herbs for salads, wraps, and other dishes.

10. Storage Containers: Invest in a variety of storage containers in different sizes to store leftovers, prepped ingredients, and homemade meals for easy grab-and-go options.

11. Herbs and Spices: Build a collection of herbs, spices, and seasonings to add flavor to your meals without relying on high-carb sauces or condiments.

12. Olive Oil and Vinegar: Keep a bottle of high-quality olive oil and vinegar on hand for dressing salads, marinating meats, and adding flavor to vegetables.

13. Low-Carb Sweeteners: Stock up on low-carb sweeteners like stevia, erythritol, or monk fruit sweetener for satisfying your sweet tooth without adding extra carbs.

14. Nuts and Seeds: Keep a variety of nuts and seeds, such as almonds, walnuts, chia seeds, and flaxseeds, for snacking, adding crunch to salads, or incorporating into recipes.

15. Low-Carb Condiments: Choose condiments like mustard, mayonnaise, hot sauce, and sugar-free ketchup to add flavor to meals without adding extra carbs.

Having these kitchen essentials on hand will help you prepare delicious, nutritious meals while following the Atkins diet, making it easier to stick to your health and wellness goals.

 - Atkins-Friendly Ingredients
Here's a list of Atkins-friendly ingredients that are suitable for women over 60 following the Atkins diet:

1. Lean Proteins:
  - Chicken breast
  - Turkey breast
  - Lean cuts of beef (e.g., sirloin, tenderloin)
  - Pork tenderloin

- Fish (e.g., salmon, tuna, cod, trout)

- Shellfish (e.g., shrimp, crab, lobster)

- Eggs

- Tofu

2. Healthy Fats:

   - Avocado

   - Olive oil

   - Coconut oil

   - Avocado oil

   - Nuts (e.g., almonds, walnuts, pecans)

   - Seeds (e.g., chia seeds, flaxseeds, pumpkin seeds)

   - Nut butters (e.g., almond butter, peanut butter)

   - Full-fat dairy products (e.g., cheese, Greek yogurt, cottage cheese)

3. Low-Carb Vegetables:

   - Leafy greens (e.g., spinach, kale, arugula, lettuce)

   - Cruciferous vegetables (e.g., broccoli, cauliflower, Brussels sprouts)

   - Zucchini

   - Cucumber

   - Bell peppers

   - Asparagus

   - Green beans

   - Mushrooms

   - Tomatoes (in moderation)

4. Herbs and Spices:

   - Basil

   - Cilantro

   - Parsley

   - Thyme

- Rosemary

- Oregano

- Garlic

- Ginger

- Turmeric

- Cumin

- Paprika

5. Low-Carb Fruits (in moderation):

   - Berries (e.g., strawberries, blueberries, raspberries)

   - Avocado

   - Tomatoes

6. Low-Carb Sweeteners:

   - Stevia

   - Erythritol

   - Monk fruit sweetener

7. Low-Carb Flours and Baking Ingredients:

   - Almond flour

   - Coconut flour

   - Flaxseed meal

   - Unsweetened cocoa powder

   - Baking powder

   - Vanilla extract

8. Low-Carb Dairy Alternatives:

   - Unsweetened almond milk

   - Unsweetened coconut milk

   - Unsweetened soy milk

9. Condiments and Sauces (choose sugar-free options):

- Mustard

- Mayonnaise

- Hot sauce

- Sugar-free ketchup

- Soy sauce (or tamari for gluten-free)

- Vinegar (e.g., apple cider vinegar, balsamic vinegar)

10. Low-Carb Snacks:

- Cheese sticks or slices

- Hard-boiled eggs

- Nuts and seeds

- Veggie sticks (e.g., cucumber, bell pepper) with dip (e.g., guacamole, hummus)

11. Fatty Fish: Incorporate fatty fish like salmon, mackerel, and sardines into your diet. These fish are rich in omega-3 fatty acids, which have anti-inflammatory properties and may support heart health, cognitive function, and joint health, which can be particularly beneficial for women over 60.

12. Bone Broth: Bone broth is a nourishing and hydrating beverage that provides essential nutrients like collagen, gelatin, and minerals. It can support gut health, joint health, and immune function, making it an excellent addition to the diet of women over 60.

13. Leafy Greens: Leafy greens such as spinach, kale, and Swiss chard are not only low in carbohydrates but also packed with vitamins, minerals, and antioxidants. They can help support bone health, eye health, and cognitive function, which are important considerations for women over 60.

14. Probiotic Foods: Include probiotic-rich foods like yogurt, kefir, sauerkraut, and kimchi in your diet to support gut health and immune function. As we age, maintaining a healthy balance

of gut bacteria becomes increasingly important for digestion, nutrient absorption, and overall well-being.

15. Collagen Powder: Collagen powder can be added to beverages or recipes to support skin health, joint health, and connective tissue function. It may help improve skin elasticity, reduce joint pain, and support mobility, which can be beneficial for women over 60.

16. Low-Carb Pasta Alternatives: Explore low-carb pasta alternatives such as zucchini noodles (zoodles), spaghetti squash, or shirataki noodles. These options allow you to enjoy pasta dishes without the high carbohydrate content, making them suitable for the Atkins diet.

17. Cauliflower Rice: Cauliflower rice is a versatile and low-carb alternative to traditional rice. It can be used as a base for stir-fries, grain bowls, or as a side dish, providing fiber, vitamins, and minerals while keeping carbohydrate intake in check.

18. Prepared Atkins Products: Consider incorporating prepared Atkins products such as shakes, bars, and frozen meals into your diet for convenience and variety. These products are specifically designed to fit within the Atkins program and can be helpful for busy lifestyles or when you need a quick and easy meal option.

   - Grocery Shopping Tips for women over 60 on the Atkins Diet

Here are some grocery shopping tips tailored for women over 60 following the Atkins Diet:

1. Plan Ahead: Before heading to the grocery store, take some time to plan your meals for the week. Look through recipes, create a shopping list, and check your pantry to see what ingredients you already have on hand.

2. Stick to the Perimeter: When navigating the grocery store, focus on shopping the perimeter where you'll find fresh produce, meats, dairy, and other whole foods. This is where you'll find the majority of Atkins-friendly ingredients.

3. Choose Fresh Produce: Opt for a variety of low-carb vegetables and fruits such as leafy greens, broccoli, cauliflower, bell peppers, berries, and avocados. These options are nutrient-dense and versatile for creating a variety of meals.

4. Select Lean Proteins: Look for lean cuts of meat, poultry, and fish. Choose skinless chicken breasts, turkey, lean cuts of beef or pork, and fatty fish like salmon or mackerel. Consider purchasing in bulk and freezing portions for later use.

5. Include Healthy Fats: Stock up on sources of healthy fats such as olive oil, avocado oil, coconut oil, nuts, seeds, and avocados. These fats are essential for satiety, nutrient absorption, and overall health.

6. Read Labels Carefully: Be mindful of reading food labels to check for hidden sugars, added carbs, and artificial ingredients. Choose products with minimal processing and natural, whole-food ingredients.

7. Consider Sugar-Free Options: Look for sugar-free or low-carb versions of condiments, sauces, and snacks. This includes items like sugar-free ketchup, mayonnaise, salad dressings, and sugar-free snacks.

8. Explore Specialty Aisles: Explore specialty sections of the grocery store, such as the natural foods or health food aisles, where you may find a wider selection of low-carb and keto-friendly products like almond flour, coconut flour, and sugar substitutes.

9. Stock up on Staples: Keep your pantry stocked with Atkins-friendly staples like canned tuna or salmon, canned vegetables (look for no-added-sugar varieties), broth or stock, herbs and spices, and low-carb baking ingredients.

10. Don't Forget Hydration: Remember to stock up on hydrating beverages like water, herbal teas, and sparkling water. Consider flavoring your water with lemon or cucumber slices for added variety.

11. Be Mindful of Portion Sizes: While shopping, keep portion sizes in mind to avoid overbuying or wasting food. Consider purchasing smaller packages or single servings of perishable items if you're concerned about consumption before expiration.

12. Budget Wisely: Plan your grocery shopping trips with your budget in mind. Look for sales, coupons, and discounts on Atkins-friendly items, and consider buying in bulk for cost savings when appropriate.

13. Choose Quality Protein Sources: Opt for high-quality protein sources that are minimally processed and free from added sugars and fillers. Look for grass-fed beef, pasture-raised poultry, and wild-caught fish whenever possible to maximize nutrient content and flavor.

14. Consider Convenience Options: While whole foods are preferable, convenience options can be helpful for busy schedules or days when you need a quick meal or snack. Look for pre-cooked proteins like rotisserie chicken, canned fish, or pre-packaged salad greens for easy meal assembly.

15. Explore Frozen Produce: Frozen vegetables and fruits can be just as nutritious as fresh and are often more convenient since they have a longer shelf life. Stock up on frozen berries, broccoli, cauliflower rice, and spinach to have on hand for quick and easy meal additions.

16. Mind Your Carb Count: Be vigilant about checking nutrition labels for carbohydrate content, especially in packaged and processed foods. Aim to choose products with no more than 5 grams of net carbs per serving to stay within the guidelines of the Atkins Diet.

17. Experiment with Low-Carb Substitutes: Get creative with low-carb substitutes for your favorite high-carb foods. Explore options like almond flour or coconut flour for baking, cauliflower rice for grains, or lettuce wraps for sandwiches and tacos.

18. Shop Seasonally: Take advantage of seasonal produce to add variety to your meals and save money. Seasonal fruits and vegetables are often fresher, tastier, and more affordable, so plan your meals around what's in season.

19. Bulk Up on Fiber: Incorporate high-fiber foods into your diet to support digestive health and promote satiety. Look for sources of soluble fiber like flaxseeds, chia seeds, and psyllium husk powder to add to smoothies, baked goods, or oatmeal.

20. Don't Forget About Electrolytes: As you transition to a lower-carb diet, you may need to pay extra attention to electrolyte balance to prevent symptoms like fatigue, headaches, or muscle cramps. Consider purchasing electrolyte supplements or consuming electrolyte-rich foods like leafy greens, avocado, and nuts.

21. Stay Flexible: While it's important to plan ahead, be flexible and open to making adjustments based on what's available at the store and your changing tastes and preferences. Don't be afraid to try new foods or recipes to keep your meals interesting and enjoyable.

- Energizing Breakfasts for women over 60

Here are some energizing breakfast ideas tailored for women over 60 on the Atkins diet:

1. Avocado and Egg Breakfast Bowl:

   - Ingredients: Avocado, eggs, cherry tomatoes, spinach, feta cheese, olive oil, salt, pepper.

   - Instructions: Mash avocado in a bowl and season with salt and pepper. Cook eggs to your liking (fried, scrambled, or poached). Serve eggs over mashed avocado with cherry tomatoes, spinach, and crumbled feta cheese. Drizzle with olive oil.

2. Greek Yogurt Parfait:

   - Ingredients: Greek yogurt (full-fat or low-fat), mixed berries (e.g., strawberries, blueberries, raspberries), unsweetened coconut flakes, almonds, chia seeds, cinnamon.

   - Instructions: Layer Greek yogurt with mixed berries in a glass or bowl. Top with unsweetened coconut flakes, sliced almonds, and a sprinkle of chia seeds and cinnamon for added flavor and texture.

3. Low-Carb Smoothie:

   - Ingredients: Unsweetened almond milk, spinach, avocado, protein powder (whey or plant-based), chia seeds, ice cubes.

   - Instructions: Blend almond milk, spinach, avocado, protein powder, and chia seeds until smooth. Add ice cubes for a refreshing texture. Customize with additional ingredients like berries, nut butter, or unsweetened cocoa powder as desired.

4. Spinach and Feta Crustless Quiche:

   - Ingredients: Eggs, spinach, feta cheese, onions, bell peppers, olive oil, salt, pepper.

   - Instructions: Preheat oven to 350°F (175°C). Sauté spinach, onions, and bell peppers in olive oil until softened. In a bowl, whisk together eggs, crumbled feta cheese, salt, and pepper. Stir in sautéed vegetables. Pour mixture into a greased pie dish and bake for 25-30 minutes, or until set and golden brown.

5. Smoked Salmon and Cream Cheese Roll-Ups:

   - Ingredients: Smoked salmon slices, cream cheese, cucumber strips, capers, lemon juice, fresh dill.

   - Instructions: Spread cream cheese on smoked salmon slices. Place cucumber strips, capers, and a squeeze of lemon juice on top. Roll up each slice and garnish with fresh dill. Serve as a refreshing and protein-packed breakfast option.

6. Coconut Flour Pancakes:

   - Ingredients: Coconut flour, eggs, unsweetened almond milk, baking powder, vanilla extract, sugar-free syrup (optional).

   - Instructions: Mix coconut flour, eggs, almond milk, baking powder, and vanilla extract until smooth. Heat a non-stick skillet over medium heat and pour batter onto the skillet to form pancakes. Cook until bubbles form on the surface, then flip and cook until golden brown. Serve with sugar-free syrup if desired.

7. Chia Seed Pudding:

   - Ingredients: Chia seeds, unsweetened almond milk, vanilla extract, sugar-free sweetener (optional), mixed berries.

   - Instructions: Mix chia seeds, almond milk, vanilla extract, and sweetener (if using) in a bowl. Let sit in the refrigerator for at least 2 hours or overnight to thicken. Serve topped with mixed berries for a nutritious and filling breakfast option.

8. Egg Muffins:

   - Ingredients: Eggs, diced vegetables (such as bell peppers, onions, spinach), cooked bacon or sausage (optional), shredded cheese (optional), salt, pepper.

   - Instructions: Preheat oven to 350°F (175°C). In a mixing bowl, whisk together eggs, diced vegetables, cooked bacon or sausage (if using), shredded cheese (if using), salt, and pepper. Pour the mixture into greased muffin tins and bake for 20-25 minutes, or until set and golden brown. These egg muffins can be made ahead of time and stored in the refrigerator for a quick grab-and-go breakfast option.

9. Low-Carb Breakfast Burrito:

   - Ingredients: Low-carb tortilla or lettuce leaves, scrambled eggs, cooked bacon or sausage, avocado slices, salsa, shredded cheese, sour cream (optional).

   - Instructions: Fill a low-carb tortilla or lettuce leaves with scrambled eggs, cooked bacon or sausage, avocado slices, salsa, shredded cheese, and sour cream if desired. Roll up the ingredients into a burrito or wrap and enjoy a satisfying and portable breakfast option.

10. Protein-Packed Omelette:

   - Ingredients: Eggs, diced vegetables (such as bell peppers, onions, mushrooms), cooked chicken or turkey breast, shredded cheese, olive oil or butter, salt, pepper, fresh herbs (such as parsley or chives).

   - Instructions: In a non-stick skillet, heat olive oil or butter over medium heat. Add diced vegetables and cooked chicken or turkey breast to the skillet and cook until softened. In a separate bowl, whisk together eggs, shredded cheese, salt, pepper, and fresh herbs. Pour the egg mixture over the cooked vegetables and meat in the skillet, swirling to evenly distribute. Cook until the omelette is set and golden brown on the bottom, then fold it over and cook for another minute or two until cooked through. Serve hot with additional toppings if desired.

11. Low-Carb Breakfast Casserole:

   - Ingredients: Eggs, diced vegetables (such as bell peppers, onions, spinach), cooked sausage or bacon, shredded cheese, heavy cream, salt, pepper.

   - Instructions: Preheat oven to 375°F (190°C). In a mixing bowl, whisk together eggs, diced vegetables, cooked sausage or bacon, shredded cheese, heavy cream, salt, and pepper. Pour the mixture into a greased baking dish and spread evenly. Bake for 30-35 minutes, or until the casserole is set and golden brown on top. Let cool slightly before slicing and serving. This breakfast casserole can be made ahead of time and reheated for quick and easy breakfasts throughout the week.

12. Vegetable Frittata:

   - Ingredients: Eggs, diced vegetables (such as bell peppers, onions, zucchini, mushrooms), olive oil, salt, pepper, fresh herbs (such as parsley or basil).

- Instructions: Preheat oven to 350°F (175°C). In an oven-safe skillet, sauté diced vegetables in olive oil until softened. In a bowl, whisk together eggs, salt, pepper, and fresh herbs. Pour the egg mixture over the sautéed vegetables in the skillet. Cook on the stovetop over medium heat until the edges begin to set, then transfer the skillet to the preheated oven and bake for 10-15 minutes, or until the frittata is cooked through and golden brown on top. Slice and serve hot.

13. Low-Carb Breakfast Tacos:
   - Ingredients: Low-carb tortillas or lettuce leaves, scrambled eggs, cooked sausage or chorizo, diced avocado, salsa, shredded cheese, cilantro.
   - Instructions: Fill low-carb tortillas or lettuce leaves with scrambled eggs, cooked sausage or chorizo, diced avocado, salsa, shredded cheese, and cilantro. Fold or roll up the tacos and enjoy a flavorful and satisfying breakfast option. Customize with additional toppings like sour cream or hot sauce as desired.

   - Low-Carb Breakfast Options
Here are some low-carb breakfast options specifically tailored for women over 60 on the Atkins diet:

1. Egg and Veggie Scramble:
   - Ingredients: Eggs, diced vegetables (such as bell peppers, onions, spinach), olive oil or butter, salt, pepper.
   - Instructions: Heat olive oil or butter in a skillet over medium heat. Add diced vegetables and sauté until softened. In a separate bowl, whisk eggs with salt and pepper. Pour the eggs into the skillet with the vegetables and scramble until cooked through. Serve hot with a side of avocado or salsa if desired.

2. Greek Yogurt with Nuts and Berries:
   - Ingredients: Greek yogurt (full-fat or low-fat), mixed nuts (such as almonds, walnuts, pecans), mixed berries (such as strawberries, blueberries, raspberries), sugar-free sweetener (optional).

- Instructions: Spoon Greek yogurt into a bowl and top with mixed nuts and berries. If desired, sprinkle with a sugar-free sweetener for added sweetness. This breakfast option is high in protein, healthy fats, and antioxidants.

3. Bacon and Avocado Wrap:
   - Ingredients: Bacon slices, avocado slices, lettuce leaves or low-carb tortilla, tomato slices, mayonnaise (optional).
   - Instructions: Cook bacon slices until crispy. Lay out lettuce leaves or a low-carb tortilla and spread with mayonnaise if desired. Layer bacon slices, avocado slices, and tomato slices on top. Roll up the wrap and enjoy a savory and satisfying breakfast.

4. Smoked Salmon and Cream Cheese Plate:
   - Ingredients: Smoked salmon slices, cream cheese, cucumber slices, capers, lemon wedges.
   - Instructions: Arrange smoked salmon slices, cream cheese, cucumber slices, and capers on a plate. Serve with lemon wedges for squeezing over the salmon. This breakfast option is low in carbs and rich in omega-3 fatty acids.

5. Low-Carb Breakfast Burrito Bowl:
   - Ingredients: Scrambled eggs, cooked sausage or chorizo, diced avocado, salsa, shredded cheese, cilantro.
   - Instructions: In a bowl, layer scrambled eggs, cooked sausage or chorizo, diced avocado, salsa, shredded cheese, and cilantro. Mix together and enjoy a flavorful breakfast bowl without the tortilla.

6. Chia Seed Pudding with Coconut Milk:
   - Ingredients: Chia seeds, unsweetened coconut milk, vanilla extract, sugar-free sweetener (optional), sliced almonds, shredded coconut.
   - Instructions: Mix chia seeds, coconut milk, vanilla extract, and sugar-free sweetener in a bowl. Let sit in the refrigerator for at least 30 minutes or overnight to thicken. Top with sliced almonds and shredded coconut before serving for added crunch and flavor.

7. Vegetable and Cheese Omelette:

- Ingredients: Eggs, diced vegetables (such as bell peppers, onions, mushrooms), shredded cheese, olive oil or butter, salt, pepper.

- Instructions: In a skillet, sauté diced vegetables in olive oil or butter until softened. In a separate bowl, whisk eggs with salt and pepper. Pour the egg mixture into the skillet with the vegetables and cook until set. Sprinkle shredded cheese on one half of the omelette and fold the other half over. Cook until the cheese is melted and serve hot.

8. Coconut Flour Pancakes:

- Ingredients: Coconut flour, eggs, unsweetened almond milk, baking powder, vanilla extract, sugar-free sweetener (optional).

- Instructions: In a mixing bowl, combine coconut flour, eggs, almond milk, baking powder, vanilla extract, and sugar-free sweetener if desired. Heat a non-stick skillet over medium heat and pour small amounts of batter onto the skillet to form pancakes. Cook until bubbles form on the surface, then flip and cook until golden brown on both sides. Serve with sugar-free syrup or fresh berries.

9. Turkey and Cheese Roll-Ups:

- Ingredients: Slices of deli turkey or chicken, cheese slices, avocado slices, mustard or mayonnaise.

- Instructions: Lay out slices of deli turkey or chicken and top each slice with a cheese slice, avocado slice, and a spread of mustard or mayonnaise. Roll up the ingredients and secure with toothpicks if necessary. Enjoy these protein-packed roll-ups as a quick and easy breakfast option.

10. Low-Carb Breakfast Hash:

- Ingredients: Diced cauliflower, diced bell peppers, diced onions, cooked bacon or sausage, eggs, shredded cheese, olive oil, salt, pepper.

- Instructions: In a skillet, heat olive oil over medium heat and add diced cauliflower, bell peppers, and onions. Cook until softened and lightly browned. Add cooked bacon or sausage to the skillet and stir to combine. Make wells in the mixture and crack eggs into each well. Cook until the eggs are set to your liking. Sprinkle with shredded cheese before serving.

11. Spinach and Mushroom Breakfast Wrap:

   - Ingredients: Low-carb tortilla or lettuce leaves, scrambled eggs, sautéed spinach, sautéed mushrooms, shredded cheese, hot sauce (optional).

   - Instructions: Fill a low-carb tortilla or lettuce leaves with scrambled eggs, sautéed spinach, sautéed mushrooms, and shredded cheese. Add hot sauce if desired. Roll up the wrap and enjoy as a flavorful and filling breakfast option.

   - Quick and Easy Morning Meals

Here are some quick and easy Atkins diet morning meal ideas for women over 60:

1. Hard-Boiled Eggs with Avocado:

   - Instructions: Simply boil a few eggs ahead of time and serve them with sliced avocado. Sprinkle with salt and pepper for added flavor. This protein-rich breakfast option is quick to prepare and provides essential nutrients to fuel your morning.

2. Low-Carb Greek Yogurt Bowl:

   - Instructions: In a bowl, combine full-fat Greek yogurt with a handful of mixed berries and a sprinkle of chopped nuts or seeds. Add a drizzle of sugar-free sweetener if desired. This breakfast is rich in protein, fiber, and healthy fats, providing a satisfying start to your day.

3. Cheese and Veggie Omelette:

   - Instructions: Whisk together eggs with diced vegetables such as bell peppers, onions, and spinach. Pour the mixture into a non-stick skillet and cook until set. Top with shredded cheese and fold the omelette in half. Serve hot for a quick and filling morning meal.

4. Protein Shake:

   - Instructions: Blend together a scoop of protein powder (whey or plant-based) with unsweetened almond milk, a handful of spinach, and a tablespoon of nut butter. Add ice cubes for a refreshing texture. This smoothie is convenient for busy mornings and provides a good balance of protein, fats, and nutrients.

5. Smoked Salmon Roll-Ups:
   - Instructions: Lay out slices of smoked salmon and spread each slice with cream cheese. Place a few cucumber slices and capers on top, then roll up the salmon slices. Enjoy these protein-rich roll-ups as a quick and portable breakfast option.

6. Low-Carb Breakfast Burrito:
   - Instructions: Fill a low-carb tortilla or lettuce leaves with scrambled eggs, cooked sausage or bacon, diced avocado, and salsa. Roll up the ingredients and enjoy a flavorful and satisfying breakfast on the go.

7. Chia Seed Pudding:
   - Instructions: Mix chia seeds with unsweetened almond milk and a splash of vanilla extract. Let the mixture sit in the refrigerator for at least 30 minutes or overnight to thicken. Top with sliced almonds and fresh berries before serving for a quick and nutritious morning meal.

8. Quick Veggie Stir-Fry:
   - Instructions: Sauté diced vegetables such as bell peppers, onions, and zucchini in olive oil until tender. Add cooked chicken or tofu for extra protein. Season with soy sauce or your favorite spices for flavor. Serve hot for a satisfying and low-carb breakfast option.

9. Low-Carb Breakfast Muffins:
   - Instructions: Mix together eggs, diced vegetables, cooked bacon or sausage, and shredded cheese. Pour the mixture into greased muffin tins and bake until set. These savory muffins can be made ahead of time and stored in the refrigerator for a quick and easy breakfast option.

10. Turkey and Cheese Roll-Ups:

- Instructions: Lay out slices of deli turkey or chicken and top each slice with a cheese slice. Roll up the slices and serve with mustard or mayonnaise for dipping. This protein-packed breakfast option is ready in minutes and perfect for busy mornings.

11. Low-Carb Breakfast Casserole Cups:

   - Instructions: Preheat your oven to 350°F (175°C). In a mixing bowl, combine beaten eggs with diced vegetables (such as bell peppers, onions, and spinach), cooked breakfast meat (such as bacon or sausage), and shredded cheese. Pour the mixture into greased muffin tins and bake for 20-25 minutes, or until set. These portable breakfast cups can be made ahead of time and stored in the refrigerator for a convenient grab-and-go option.

12. Cottage Cheese with Berries and Almonds:

   - Instructions: Spoon full-fat cottage cheese into a bowl and top with mixed berries (such as strawberries, blueberries, and raspberries) and a handful of almonds. Drizzle with a touch of sugar-free sweetener or a sprinkle of cinnamon for added flavor. This quick and easy breakfast option is rich in protein and healthy fats to keep you feeling satisfied.

13. Quick Avocado Toast:

   - Instructions: Toast a slice of low-carb bread or a whole grain English muffin. Mash half an avocado and spread it onto the toast. Top with sliced tomatoes, a sprinkle of salt and pepper, and a drizzle of olive oil or hot sauce if desired. This savory breakfast option is ready in minutes and provides a good balance of nutrients to start your day.

14. Low-Carb Breakfast Wrap:

   - Instructions: Lay out a low-carb tortilla or large lettuce leaves and fill them with scrambled eggs, cooked bacon or sausage, diced avocado, and shredded cheese. Roll up the wrap and enjoy a delicious and satisfying breakfast on the go. Customize with your favorite toppings such as salsa or sour cream for added flavor.

15. Quick Protein Pancakes:

- Instructions: In a mixing bowl, whisk together eggs, protein powder (whey or plant-based), and a splash of unsweetened almond milk until smooth. Heat a non-stick skillet over medium heat and pour small amounts of batter onto the skillet to form pancakes. Cook until bubbles form on the surface, then flip and cook until golden brown on both sides. Serve with a dollop of Greek yogurt and fresh berries for a protein-packed breakfast option.

16. Microwave Egg Mug:

   - Instructions: Crack an egg into a microwave-safe mug and whisk it with a fork. Add diced vegetables, shredded cheese, and cooked bacon or sausage if desired. Microwave on high for 1-2 minutes, or until the egg is set. Enjoy this quick and easy breakfast option straight from the mug or slide it onto a plate for serving.

17. Quick Greek Yogurt Parfait:

   - Instructions: In a glass or bowl, layer full-fat Greek yogurt with low-carb granola or crushed nuts and mixed berries. Repeat the layers until the glass or bowl is filled. Drizzle with a touch of sugar-free syrup or honey for added sweetness if desired. This simple breakfast parfait is ready in minutes and provides a good balance of protein, fiber, and antioxidants.

18. Low-Carb Breakfast Smoothie:

   - Instructions: Blend together unsweetened almond milk, spinach, frozen berries, protein powder (whey or plant-based), and a tablespoon of nut butter until smooth. Add ice cubes for a refreshing texture. Pour into a glass and enjoy this nutrient-packed breakfast smoothie on the go.

- Healthy and Filling Lunch Ideas

Creating healthy and filling lunch ideas for women over 60 on the Atkins diet requires a balance of nutritious ingredients while keeping carbohydrate intake low. Here are some ideas:

1. Grilled Chicken Salad: Start with a base of mixed greens and add grilled chicken breast slices. Top with sliced cucumbers, cherry tomatoes, avocado, and feta cheese. Dress with olive oil and vinegar or a low-carb vinaigrette.

2. Turkey Lettuce Wraps: Use large lettuce leaves as wraps and fill them with sliced turkey breast, sliced cheese, avocado, and mustard or mayo. Add a side of raw veggies like bell pepper strips or celery sticks for extra crunch.

3. Cauliflower Rice Stir-Fry: Sauté cauliflower rice with mixed vegetables like bell peppers, broccoli, and snap peas in olive oil. Add cooked shrimp or tofu for protein, and season with soy sauce, garlic, and ginger for flavor.

4. Egg Salad Lettuce Cups: Make egg salad using hard-boiled eggs, mayo, mustard, and diced celery. Serve scoops of egg salad in large lettuce leaves. Add a side of sliced cucumbers and radishes for freshness.

5. Zucchini Noodles with Pesto and Chicken: Spiralize zucchini into noodles and sauté them in olive oil until tender. Toss with homemade or store-bought pesto sauce and grilled chicken strips. Sprinkle with grated Parmesan cheese.

6. Tuna Salad Stuffed Avocado: Mix canned tuna with mayo, diced onions, and celery. Cut avocados in half and remove the pit, then fill the avocado halves with the tuna salad mixture. Serve with a side of mixed greens dressed with olive oil and lemon juice.

7. Salmon and Asparagus Foil Packets: Season salmon fillets with lemon juice, olive oil, and herbs. Place each fillet on a piece of foil along with asparagus spears. Seal the foil packets and bake or grill until the salmon is cooked through.

8. Greek Yogurt Chicken Salad: Combine cooked diced chicken breast with Greek yogurt, diced cucumber, red onion, dill, and lemon juice. Serve on a bed of mixed greens with sliced tomatoes and olives.

9. Stuffed Bell Peppers: Cut bell peppers in half and remove the seeds. Fill them with a mixture of cooked ground turkey or chicken, cauliflower rice, diced tomatoes, onions, and spices. Top with shredded cheese and bake until the peppers are tender and the filling is heated through.

10. Cobb Salad: Create a Cobb salad with mixed greens as the base and top with sliced hard-boiled eggs, grilled chicken breast strips, crumbled bacon, avocado slices, and blue cheese crumbles. Drizzle with a creamy low-carb dressing, such as ranch or blue cheese.

11. Eggplant Parmesan: Make a lighter version of eggplant Parmesan by layering thinly sliced eggplant with marinara sauce and mozzarella cheese. Bake until the eggplant is tender and the cheese is bubbly. Serve with a side salad dressed with olive oil and vinegar.

12. Shrimp and Avocado Salad: Combine cooked shrimp with diced avocado, cucumber, red onion, and cilantro. Toss with lime juice, olive oil, and a pinch of salt and pepper. Serve over mixed greens for a refreshing and satisfying salad.

13. Zucchini Boats: Cut zucchini in half lengthwise and scoop out the seeds to create "boats." Fill the boats with a mixture of cooked ground beef or turkey, diced tomatoes, onions, bell peppers, and spices. Top with shredded cheese and bake until the zucchini is tender.

14. Chicken Caesar Salad: Toss grilled chicken breast slices with romaine lettuce, Parmesan cheese, and Caesar dressing (opt for a low-carb version or make your own with olive oil, anchovies, garlic, and lemon juice). Add some cherry tomatoes and crispy bacon for extra flavor.

15. Tofu Stir-Fry: Cube tofu and stir-fry it with mixed vegetables like broccoli, bell peppers, mushrooms, and snap peas. Season with soy sauce, garlic, ginger, and a splash of sesame oil. Serve over cauliflower rice for a low-carb twist.

16. Greek Chicken Wrap: Fill a low-carb tortilla or large lettuce leaves with grilled chicken strips, diced tomatoes, cucumbers, red onion, olives, and feta cheese. Drizzle with tzatziki sauce or a Greek yogurt-based dressing for extra flavor.

17. Salmon Salad: Flake cooked salmon and toss with mixed greens, sliced cucumber, cherry tomatoes, and avocado. Dress with a lemon-dill vinaigrette made with olive oil, lemon juice, fresh dill, salt, and pepper.

18. Stuffed Portobello Mushrooms: Remove the stems from portobello mushrooms and brush them with olive oil. Fill the caps with a mixture of cooked spinach, ricotta cheese, garlic, and herbs. Bake until the mushrooms are tender and the filling is heated through.

19. **Tuna Stuffed Cucumbers**: Mix canned tuna with Greek yogurt or mayonnaise, diced celery, and seasonings like dill, lemon juice, and black pepper. Slice cucumbers in half lengthwise and scoop out the seeds to create a "boat." Fill the cucumber halves with the tuna mixture for a crunchy and satisfying lunch.

20. Turkey and Veggie Roll-Ups: Lay slices of turkey breast flat and spread them with cream cheese or avocado spread. Add strips of bell peppers, cucumber, and spinach leaves. Roll up the turkey slices and secure with toothpicks for a portable and low-carb lunch option.

21. Mushroom and Spinach Omelette: Cook sliced mushrooms and spinach in a non-stick skillet until wilted. Pour beaten eggs seasoned with salt and pepper over the vegetables and cook until set. Fold the omelette in half and serve with a side salad for a nutritious and protein-packed meal.

22. Cauliflower Crust Pizza: Make a pizza crust using cauliflower rice, eggs, shredded cheese, and seasonings. Top the crust with sugar-free marinara sauce, sliced veggies like bell peppers and onions, and cooked chicken or turkey sausage. Bake until the crust is crispy and the toppings are bubbly.

23. Salami and Cheese Platter: Arrange slices of salami, cheese, and olives on a plate. Add cherry tomatoes, cucumber slices, and pickles for extra variety. Serve with mustard or a low-carb dip for a satisfying and effortless lunch.

24. Stuffed Chicken Breast: Flatten chicken breast fillets and stuff them with a mixture of spinach, sun-dried tomatoes, and goat cheese. Roll up the chicken and secure with toothpicks. Bake until the chicken is cooked through and the filling is bubbly and golden brown.

25. Cabbage and Beef Stir-Fry: Thinly slice cabbage and stir-fry it with ground beef or turkey, garlic, ginger, and soy sauce. Add in sliced bell peppers, carrots, and snap peas for extra crunch and flavor. Serve hot for a hearty and nutritious meal.

26. Broccoli Cheddar Soup: Make a creamy broccoli cheddar soup using pureed steamed broccoli, chicken broth, heavy cream, and shredded cheddar cheese. Season with salt, pepper, and a pinch of nutmeg for extra flavor. Serve with a side salad or low-carb crackers.

27. Shrimp Caesar Salad: Grill or sauté shrimp seasoned with garlic and lemon juice until cooked through. Toss with romaine lettuce, Parmesan cheese, and Caesar dressing. Add crispy bacon bits and croutons made from low-carb bread for extra texture.

28. Caprese Stuffed Avocado: Halve avocados and remove the pits. Fill the avocado halves with cherry tomatoes, fresh mozzarella cheese balls, and basil leaves. Drizzle with balsamic glaze and sprinkle with salt and pepper for a simple yet flavorful lunch option.

- Portable Lunch Options for women over 60

Here are some portable lunch options that are convenient for women over 60 following the Atkins diet:

1. Egg Muffins: Make mini egg muffins by whisking eggs with diced vegetables like bell peppers, spinach, and mushrooms. Pour the mixture into greased muffin tins and bake until set. These portable egg muffins can be enjoyed hot or cold and make a great on-the-go lunch option.

2. Cheese and Nut Snack Box: Pack a variety of cheese cubes, such as cheddar, mozzarella, and Swiss, along with a handful of mixed nuts like almonds, walnuts, and pecans. Add some cherry tomatoes, cucumber slices, and olives for extra flavor and freshness.

3. Chicken Salad Lettuce Wraps: Prepare a batch of chicken salad using diced cooked chicken, mayo, diced celery, and seasonings. Spoon the chicken salad into large lettuce leaves and wrap them up for a low-carb and portable lunch option.

4. Salmon Cucumber Bites: Top cucumber slices with smoked salmon, cream cheese, and fresh dill for a light and refreshing snack. These bite-sized treats are perfect for a midday pick-me-up and can be easily packed in a lunchbox or cooler.

5. Veggie and Hummus Cups: Pack small containers with hummus and sliced vegetables like bell peppers, carrots, and celery sticks. The combination of crunchy veggies and creamy hummus makes for a satisfying and nutritious portable snack.

6. Turkey and Cheese Roll-Ups: Roll slices of deli turkey around cheese sticks or slices. Add a smear of mustard or mayo for extra flavor, then secure the roll-ups with toothpicks. These protein-packed snacks are easy to eat on the go and can be customized with your favorite cheese varieties.

7. Tuna Cucumber Boats: Scoop out the seeds from cucumber halves to create "boats." Fill the cucumber halves with tuna salad made from canned tuna, mayo, diced onions, and seasonings. These refreshing cucumber boats are perfect for a light and portable lunch option.

8. Greek Yogurt Parfait: Layer Greek yogurt with mixed berries, nuts, and seeds in a portable container. Greek yogurt is high in protein and low in carbs, making it an ideal choice for those following the Atkins diet. Customize your parfait with your favorite toppings for a delicious and satisfying snack.

9. Avocado and Bacon Stuffed Cherry Tomatoes: Halve cherry tomatoes and scoop out the seeds. Fill the tomato halves with mashed avocado and top with crispy bacon bits. These bite-sized snacks are packed with flavor and healthy fats, making them a great portable option for a quick lunch or snack.

10. Protein Bars or Shakes: Keep a stash of low-carb protein bars or shakes on hand for busy days when you need a quick and convenient meal replacement. Look for options with minimal added sugars and ingredients that fit within the Atkins diet guidelines.

11. Sliced Veggie and Turkey Wraps: Spread a thin layer of cream cheese or avocado spread on deli turkey slices. Place a few strips of bell peppers, cucumber, and carrot on each slice, then roll them up. Secure the wraps with toothpicks and pack them for an easy and low-carb lunch.

12. Cauliflower and Broccoli Salad: Make a salad with steamed cauliflower and broccoli florets tossed with diced red onion, crispy bacon bits, and shredded cheddar cheese. Dress the salad with a creamy low-carb dressing, such as ranch or blue cheese, for a satisfying and portable meal.

13. Salami and Cream Cheese Roll-Ups: Spread cream cheese on slices of salami and top with a sprinkle of chopped fresh herbs like parsley or chives. Roll up the salami slices and secure them with toothpicks for a savory and portable snack that's perfect for on-the-go.

14. Prosciutto-Wrapped Asparagus Spears: Wrap blanched asparagus spears with thin slices of prosciutto for a simple and elegant snack. The combination of salty prosciutto and tender asparagus is sure to satisfy your cravings while keeping you on track with your low-carb diet.

15. Beef Jerky and Cheese Sticks: Pack individual portions of beef jerky and cheese sticks for a convenient and protein-rich snack. Look for beef jerky options with minimal added sugars and preservatives, and choose cheese sticks made from real cheese for the best nutritional value.

16. Mozzarella and Tomato Skewers: Thread cherry tomatoes and bite-sized mozzarella cheese balls onto wooden skewers for a portable and delicious snack. Drizzle the skewers with balsamic glaze and sprinkle with fresh basil leaves for added flavor.

17. Smoked Salmon and Cream Cheese Cucumber Rounds: Slice cucumbers into rounds and spread each round with cream cheese. Top with smoked salmon and a sprinkle of capers for a sophisticated and low-carb snack that's perfect for entertaining or enjoying on the go.

18. Almond Butter and Celery Sticks: Spread almond butter on celery sticks for a crunchy and satisfying snack that's rich in healthy fats and protein. Add a sprinkle of cinnamon or a drizzle of honey for extra flavor, if desired.

19. Parmesan Crisps: Bake grated Parmesan cheese in the oven until crispy and golden brown for a crunchy and low-carb snack. These homemade Parmesan crisps are perfect for munching on when you need a quick and satisfying pick-me-up.

20. Greek Salad Skewers: Thread cherry tomatoes, cucumber slices, feta cheese cubes, and Kalamata olives onto wooden skewers for a portable and flavorful snack inspired by classic Greek salad flavors.

  - Salads, Soups, and Sandwiches

Here are some salad, soup, and sandwich ideas tailored for women over 60 following the Atkins diet:

Salads:

1. Grilled Chicken Caesar Salad: Toss grilled chicken breast slices with romaine lettuce, Parmesan cheese, and a creamy Caesar dressing made with mayonnaise, anchovies, garlic, and lemon juice. Add crispy bacon bits and croutons made from low-carb bread for extra flavor and crunch.

2. Greek Salad: Combine mixed greens with cherry tomatoes, cucumber slices, Kalamata olives, red onion, and feta cheese. Dress the salad with olive oil, lemon juice, oregano, salt, and pepper for a refreshing and flavorful dish.

3. Tuna Nicoise Salad: Arrange mixed greens on a plate and top with canned tuna, boiled eggs, green beans, cherry tomatoes, olives, and boiled potatoes (optional). Drizzle with a Dijon vinaigrette made with olive oil, red wine vinegar, Dijon mustard, and minced shallots.

4. Cobb Salad: Create a Cobb salad with mixed greens as the base and top with sliced hard-boiled eggs, grilled chicken breast strips, crumbled bacon, avocado slices, and blue cheese crumbles. Drizzle with a creamy low-carb dressing, such as ranch or blue cheese.

5. Caprese Salad: Layer sliced tomatoes, fresh mozzarella cheese, and basil leaves on a plate. Drizzle with balsamic glaze and extra virgin olive oil, and sprinkle with salt and pepper for a simple yet elegant salad.

Soups:

1. Creamy Broccoli Soup: Puree steamed broccoli with chicken broth, heavy cream, and grated cheddar cheese until smooth. Season with salt, pepper, and a pinch of nutmeg for a comforting and creamy soup that's low in carbs.

2. Tomato Basil Soup: Simmer canned tomatoes with onion, garlic, chicken broth, and fresh basil until the flavors meld together. Puree the soup until smooth, then stir in heavy cream for richness. Serve hot with a sprinkle of Parmesan cheese on top.

3. Chicken and Vegetable Soup: Make a hearty soup with diced chicken breast, mixed vegetables like celery, carrots, and bell peppers, and chicken broth. Season with herbs like thyme and rosemary for added flavor, and simmer until the chicken is cooked through and the vegetables are tender.

4. Egg Drop Soup: Bring chicken broth to a simmer and slowly pour beaten eggs into the broth while stirring gently to create ribbons of cooked egg. Season with soy sauce, sesame oil, and green onions for a simple and comforting soup option.

5. Mexican Chicken Tortilla Soup: Simmer shredded chicken breast with diced tomatoes, bell peppers, onions, and spices like cumin, chili powder, and paprika in chicken broth. Serve the soup hot with avocado slices, shredded cheese, and crushed pork rinds as a low-carb alternative to tortilla strips.

Sandwiches:

1. Lettuce-Wrapped Burger: Grill or pan-sear a burger patty and wrap it in large lettuce leaves instead of a bun. Top the burger with sliced tomato, red onion, and avocado, and add a smear of mustard or mayo for extra flavor.

2. Turkey and Avocado Wrap: Spread mashed avocado on a low-carb tortilla or large lettuce leaves and top with sliced turkey breast, bacon, lettuce, and tomato. Roll up the wrap and secure it with toothpicks for a satisfying and portable lunch option.

3. Egg Salad Sandwich: Make egg salad with hard-boiled eggs, mayo, mustard, and diced celery. Spread the egg salad on low-carb bread or lettuce leaves and add sliced cucumber and sprouts for extra crunch.

4. Tuna Melt: Mix canned tuna with mayo, diced onions, and celery, and spread it on low-carb bread slices. Top with sliced tomato and shredded cheese, then broil until the cheese is melted and bubbly for a comforting and satisfying sandwich option.

5. BLT Wrap: Fill a low-carb tortilla or large lettuce leaves with crispy bacon, sliced tomato, and lettuce. Add a smear of mayo or avocado spread for extra creaminess, then roll up the wrap for a classic and delicious lunch option.

<u>**Chapter 6. Dinner Recipes**</u>

- Nutritious Dinners for women over 60

Here are some nutritious dinner ideas specifically designed for women over 60 following the Atkins diet:

1. Grilled Salmon with Roasted Vegetables: Grill salmon fillets seasoned with lemon, garlic, and herbs until cooked through. Serve with a side of roasted low-carb vegetables such as cauliflower, Brussels sprouts, and asparagus tossed in olive oil and seasoned with salt and pepper.

2. Baked Chicken Thighs with Cauliflower Mash: Season chicken thighs with your favorite herbs and spices, then bake until golden and cooked through. Pair the chicken with creamy mashed cauliflower made with butter, heavy cream, and garlic for a satisfying and low-carb alternative to mashed potatoes.

3. Stuffed Bell Peppers with Ground Beef and Cheese: Hollow out bell peppers and fill them with a mixture of cooked ground beef, diced tomatoes, onions, and shredded cheese. Bake until the peppers are tender and the filling is bubbly and golden brown for a flavorful and satisfying dinner option.

4. Zucchini Noodles with Pesto and Grilled Shrimp: Spiralize zucchini into noodles and sauté them in olive oil until tender. Toss the zucchini noodles with homemade or store-bought pesto sauce and grilled shrimp for a light and refreshing meal that's full of flavor.

5. Baked Turkey Meatballs with Marinara Sauce: Mix ground turkey with almond flour, Parmesan cheese, eggs, and seasonings to make meatballs. Bake the meatballs until cooked through, then serve with low-carb marinara sauce and a side salad for a classic and satisfying dinner option.

6. Stir-Fried Beef and Broccoli: Stir-fry thinly sliced beef with broccoli florets, bell peppers, and onions in a mixture of soy sauce, garlic, and ginger. Serve the stir-fry over cauliflower rice for a low-carb twist on this classic dish.

7. Eggplant Lasagna: Layer thinly sliced eggplant with marinara sauce, ricotta cheese, and mozzarella cheese in a baking dish. Bake until the eggplant is tender and the cheese is bubbly and golden brown for a delicious and low-carb alternative to traditional lasagna.

8. Baked Cod with Lemon and Herbs: Season cod fillets with lemon zest, garlic, and fresh herbs like parsley and thyme. Bake the cod until flaky and cooked through, then serve with a side of steamed green beans or roasted Brussels sprouts for a light and nutritious dinner option.

9. Cauliflower Crust Pizza with Veggie Toppings: Make a pizza crust using cauliflower rice, eggs, and shredded cheese, then top it with sugar-free marinara sauce, sliced vegetables like bell peppers and mushrooms, and cooked chicken or turkey sausage. Bake until the crust is crispy and the toppings are bubbly for a delicious and low-carb pizza option.

10. Grilled Steak with Creamed Spinach: Grill steak to your desired doneness and serve it with a side of creamed spinach made with sautéed spinach, cream cheese, heavy cream, and garlic. This hearty and satisfying meal is perfect for a special occasion or weeknight dinner.

11. Stuffed Portobello Mushrooms: Remove the stems from portobello mushrooms and brush them with olive oil. Fill the caps with a mixture of cooked spinach, ricotta cheese, garlic, and herbs. Top with grated Parmesan cheese and bake until the mushrooms are tender and the filling is heated through.

12. Cabbage Roll Casserole: Brown ground beef or turkey with onions, garlic, and Italian seasoning. Layer the meat mixture with shredded cabbage in a baking dish, then top with low-carb marinara sauce and shredded mozzarella cheese. Bake until bubbly and golden brown for a hearty and comforting dinner option.

13. Coconut Curry Chicken: Sauté diced chicken breast with onions, bell peppers, and cauliflower in a coconut milk-based curry sauce flavored with ginger, garlic, and curry powder. Serve the curry over cauliflower rice for a flavorful and satisfying meal.

14. Baked Pork Chops with Roasted Brussels Sprouts: Season pork chops with salt, pepper, and your favorite herbs, then bake until cooked through. Serve the pork chops with roasted Brussels sprouts tossed in olive oil and seasoned with garlic powder, paprika, and Parmesan cheese for a simple and nutritious dinner option.

15. Shrimp and Avocado Salad: Combine cooked shrimp with diced avocado, cucumber, red onion, and cilantro. Toss with lime juice, olive oil, and a pinch of salt and pepper. Serve over mixed greens for a refreshing and protein-packed salad that's perfect for a light dinner.

16. Turkey and Vegetable Stir-Fry: Stir-fry sliced turkey breast with mixed vegetables like bell peppers, broccoli, and snap peas in a mixture of soy sauce, garlic, and ginger. Serve the stir-fry over cauliflower rice for a low-carb and satisfying meal that's quick and easy to make.

17. Mushroom and Spinach Quiche: Line a pie dish with a low-carb crust or use a crustless quiche base made with eggs and heavy cream. Fill the quiche with sautéed mushrooms, spinach, and shredded cheese, then bake until set for a flavorful and protein-packed dinner option.

18. Grilled Lemon Herb Chicken Kabobs: Marinate chunks of chicken breast in a mixture of lemon juice, olive oil, garlic, and herbs like rosemary and thyme. Thread the marinated chicken onto skewers with bell peppers, onions, and cherry tomatoes, then grill until the chicken is cooked through and the vegetables are tender.

19. Sausage and Cauliflower Casserole: Brown sausage in a skillet with onions and garlic, then combine with cooked cauliflower florets in a baking dish. Top with shredded cheese and bake until bubbly and golden brown for a hearty and comforting dinner option.

20. Salmon with Dill Cream Sauce: Pan-sear or bake salmon fillets until cooked through, then serve with a creamy dill sauce made with Greek yogurt, lemon juice, and fresh dill. Pair the salmon with steamed or roasted vegetables for a nutritious and delicious dinner.

- One-Pot Meals for Easy Cleanup

One-pot meals are not only convenient for easy cleanup but also perfect for women over 60 on the Atkins diet. Here are some delicious and low-carb one-pot meal ideas:

1. Cauliflower Chicken Alfredo: Cook diced chicken breast in a skillet with garlic and olive oil until browned. Add cauliflower florets and chicken broth to the skillet and simmer until the cauliflower is tender. Stir in heavy cream and grated Parmesan cheese until the sauce is creamy and thickened. Season with salt, pepper, and nutmeg, then serve hot.

2. Sausage and Vegetable Skillet: Brown sliced sausage in a skillet with onions and bell peppers until cooked through. Add diced zucchini, cherry tomatoes, and spinach to the skillet and cook until the vegetables are tender. Season with Italian herbs, garlic powder, and red pepper flakes for extra flavor.

3. Shrimp Cauliflower Fried Rice: Sauté shrimp in a skillet with garlic and ginger until pink and cooked through. Remove the shrimp from the skillet and set aside. Add riced cauliflower, diced carrots, peas, and green onions to the skillet and cook until the cauliflower is tender. Push the cauliflower mixture to one side of the skillet and scramble eggs on the other side. Stir everything together, then add the cooked shrimp back to the skillet and toss to combine. Season with soy sauce and sesame oil, then serve hot.

4. Beef and Broccoli Stir-Fry: Stir-fry thinly sliced beef with broccoli florets, sliced bell peppers, and onions in a skillet with garlic and ginger until the beef is browned and the vegetables are tender-crisp. Add soy sauce and sesame oil to the skillet and toss to coat. Serve hot over cauliflower rice for a low-carb and satisfying meal.

5. Creamy Tuscan Chicken: Brown chicken thighs in a skillet with olive oil until golden and cooked through. Remove the chicken from the skillet and set aside. Add sliced mushrooms, sun-dried tomatoes, and spinach to the skillet and cook until the vegetables are wilted. Stir in heavy cream and grated Parmesan cheese until the sauce is creamy and thickened. Return the

chicken to the skillet and simmer until heated through. Serve hot with a sprinkle of fresh parsley on top.

6. Spaghetti Squash Carbonara: Cook spaghetti squash in the microwave or oven until tender. Meanwhile, sauté diced pancetta or bacon in a skillet until crispy. Add minced garlic to the skillet and cook until fragrant. Add cooked spaghetti squash to the skillet along with beaten eggs and grated Parmesan cheese. Stir everything together until the eggs are cooked and the sauce is creamy. Season with black pepper and chopped parsley before serving.

7. Mexican Cauliflower Rice Casserole: Cook ground beef with onions, garlic, and taco seasoning in a skillet until browned. Stir in riced cauliflower, diced tomatoes, chopped green chilies, and shredded cheese. Transfer the mixture to a baking dish and bake until bubbly and golden brown. Serve hot with toppings like avocado, sour cream, and chopped cilantro.

8. Lemon Garlic Shrimp and Asparagus: Sauté shrimp in a skillet with garlic, lemon zest, and red pepper flakes until pink and cooked through. Remove the shrimp from the skillet and set aside. Add trimmed asparagus spears to the skillet and cook until crisp-tender. Return the shrimp to the skillet and toss to combine. Serve hot with a squeeze of lemon juice on top.

9. Creamy Mushroom and Spinach Chicken: Brown chicken breasts in a skillet with olive oil until golden and cooked through. Remove the chicken from the skillet and set aside. Add sliced mushrooms and minced garlic to the skillet and cook until the mushrooms are browned. Stir in heavy cream and chopped spinach until the sauce is creamy and thickened. Return the chicken to the skillet and simmer until heated through. Serve hot with a sprinkle of grated Parmesan cheese on top.

10. Zucchini Noodle Primavera: Sauté diced onion, bell pepper, and cherry tomatoes in a skillet with garlic and olive oil until tender. Add spiralized zucchini noodles to the skillet and cook until al dente. Stir in cooked shrimp or grilled chicken strips until heated through. Season with Italian herbs, salt, and pepper before serving.

11. Egg Roll in a Bowl: Brown ground pork or turkey in a large skillet with minced garlic, ginger, and soy sauce until cooked through. Add shredded cabbage, carrots, and sliced bell peppers to the skillet and cook until the vegetables are tender-crisp. Stir in chopped green onions and sesame oil, then serve hot for a low-carb and flavorful meal.

12. Lemon Herb Baked Cod with Vegetables: Place cod fillets on a baking sheet and season with lemon zest, minced garlic, and chopped fresh herbs like parsley and thyme. Arrange mixed vegetables such as cherry tomatoes, zucchini slices, and green beans around the fish. Drizzle everything with olive oil and lemon juice, then bake until the fish is flaky and the vegetables are tender.

13. Sausage and Kale Soup: Brown sliced sausage in a large pot with onions, garlic, and Italian seasoning until cooked through. Add chopped kale, diced tomatoes, chicken broth, and cannellini beans to the pot and simmer until the kale is wilted and tender. Season with salt, pepper, and red pepper flakes for a hearty and comforting soup option.

14. Pesto Chicken and Vegetable Skillet: Sauté diced chicken breast in a skillet with olive oil until browned and cooked through. Add sliced mushrooms, diced zucchini, and halved cherry tomatoes to the skillet and cook until the vegetables are tender. Stir in pesto sauce and heavy cream until heated through, then serve hot with a sprinkle of grated Parmesan cheese on top.

15. Beef and Cabbage Stir-Fry: Brown ground beef in a large skillet with minced garlic, ginger, and soy sauce until cooked through. Add shredded cabbage, sliced bell peppers, and diced onions to the skillet and cook until the vegetables are tender-crisp. Serve hot over cauliflower rice for a low-carb and satisfying meal.

16. Creamy Tuscan Shrimp Pasta: Sauté shrimp in a large skillet with olive oil, minced garlic, and sun-dried tomatoes until pink and cooked through. Remove the shrimp from the skillet and set aside. Add chopped spinach and diced artichoke hearts to the skillet and cook until the spinach is wilted. Stir in heavy cream and grated Parmesan cheese until the sauce is creamy and

thickened. Return the shrimp to the skillet and simmer until heated through. Serve hot over zucchini noodles or spaghetti squash for a low-carb twist on this classic dish.

17. Mushroom and Spinach Quinoa Pilaf: Sauté sliced mushrooms and minced garlic in a large pot with olive oil until browned. Add rinsed quinoa and chicken broth to the pot and bring to a boil. Reduce heat, cover, and simmer until the quinoa is cooked and fluffy. Stir in chopped spinach until wilted, then serve hot as a nutritious and satisfying side dish or vegetarian main course.

18. Buffalo Chicken Cauliflower Casserole: Cook diced chicken breast in a skillet with buffalo sauce until cooked through. In a large baking dish, layer cooked cauliflower florets with the buffalo chicken mixture and shredded cheese. Bake until bubbly and golden brown for a spicy and satisfying low-carb casserole option.

19. Italian Sausage and Peppers with Cauliflower Rice: Brown sliced Italian sausage in a large skillet with sliced bell peppers and onions until cooked through. Serve the sausage and peppers over cauliflower rice cooked with minced garlic and Italian seasoning for a flavorful and low-carb twist on this classic dish.

20. Zucchini Lasagna: Layer sliced zucchini, marinara sauce, ricotta cheese, and shredded mozzarella cheese in a large baking dish. Repeat the layers until the dish is filled, then bake until bubbly and golden brown for a delicious and low-carb alternative to traditional lasagna.

These one-pot meal ideas are not only easy to prepare but also provide plenty of flavor and nutrition for women over 60 following the Atkins diet. Plus, with only one pot to clean, they make cleanup a breeze!.

 - Flavorful Main Dishes without the Carbs

Here are some flavorful main dishes without the carbs that are perfect for women over 60 on the Atkins diet:

1. Grilled Lemon Herb Chicken: Marinate chicken breasts in a mixture of lemon juice, olive oil, minced garlic, and chopped herbs like rosemary, thyme, and parsley. Grill until cooked through and serve with a squeeze of fresh lemon juice for added flavor.

2. Baked Salmon with Dill Butter: Season salmon fillets with salt, pepper, and lemon zest, then bake until flaky and tender. While the salmon is baking, melt butter with minced garlic and chopped fresh dill in a small saucepan. Drizzle the dill butter over the baked salmon just before serving for a burst of flavor.

3. Garlic Butter Steak: Sear steaks in a hot skillet with melted butter and minced garlic until browned and cooked to your desired doneness. Let the steaks rest before slicing, then drizzle with the garlic butter pan sauce for extra flavor.

4. Shrimp Scampi: Sauté shrimp in a skillet with melted butter, minced garlic, lemon zest, and white wine until pink and cooked through. Serve over zucchini noodles or spaghetti squash for a low-carb twist on this classic dish.

5. Lemon Rosemary Roast Chicken: Rub a whole chicken with olive oil, lemon zest, minced garlic, and chopped fresh rosemary. Roast in the oven until golden and crispy on the outside and tender and juicy on the inside for a flavorful and comforting main dish.

6. Pesto Baked Cod: Spread pesto sauce over cod fillets and bake until flaky and cooked through. Serve with a squeeze of fresh lemon juice and a sprinkle of grated Parmesan cheese for a burst of flavor.

7. Cajun Grilled Shrimp: Toss shrimp in Cajun seasoning and olive oil, then grill until pink and cooked through. Serve with a squeeze of fresh lime juice and a sprinkle of chopped cilantro for a zesty and flavorful main dish.

8. Herb Roasted Pork Tenderloin: Rub pork tenderloin with a mixture of chopped herbs like thyme, rosemary, and sage, along with minced garlic and olive oil. Roast in the oven until cooked through and serve with a side of low-carb vegetables for a hearty and flavorful meal.

9. Chimichurri Steak: Grill steak to your desired doneness, then top with homemade chimichurri sauce made with fresh parsley, cilantro, garlic, red wine vinegar, and olive oil. Serve hot with a side of grilled vegetables for a delicious and low-carb main dish.

10. Greek Lemon Garlic Chicken Skewers: Marinate chicken breast cubes in a mixture of lemon juice, minced garlic, dried oregano, and olive oil. Thread onto skewers and grill until cooked through. Serve with a side of Greek yogurt tzatziki sauce for dipping and a Greek salad for a complete and flavorful meal.

11. Thai Coconut Curry Shrimp: Sauté shrimp in a skillet with red curry paste, coconut milk, minced garlic, and chopped ginger until cooked through. Stir in sliced bell peppers, bamboo shoots, and snow peas, then simmer until the vegetables are tender. Serve hot over cauliflower rice for a flavorful and satisfying meal.

12. Mediterranean Baked Chicken: Season chicken thighs with a mixture of dried herbs like oregano, thyme, and basil, along with minced garlic and lemon zest. Bake until golden and crispy on the outside and juicy on the inside. Serve with a side of Greek salad and tzatziki sauce for a refreshing and flavorful dinner option.

13. Italian Stuffed Bell Peppers: Hollow out bell peppers and fill them with a mixture of cooked ground beef or turkey, diced tomatoes, minced garlic, Italian seasoning, and grated Parmesan cheese. Bake until the peppers are tender and the filling is heated through for a hearty and flavorful main dish.

14. Sesame Ginger Tofu Stir-Fry: Marinate cubed tofu in a mixture of soy sauce, minced ginger, sesame oil, and rice vinegar for at least 30 minutes. Stir-fry the marinated tofu in a skillet with

sliced bell peppers, broccoli florets, and snap peas until the vegetables are tender-crisp. Serve hot over cauliflower rice for a satisfying and flavorful vegetarian option.

15. Garlic Herb Butter Baked Halibut: Season halibut fillets with salt, pepper, and a mixture of minced garlic, chopped parsley, and melted butter. Bake until flaky and cooked through, then serve with a squeeze of fresh lemon juice for a simple yet flavorful main dish.

16. Indian Spiced Lamb Chops: Rub lamb chops with a mixture of garam masala, ground cumin, ground coriander, minced garlic, and olive oil. Grill or pan-sear until cooked to your desired doneness, then serve hot with a side of cucumber raita and steamed cauliflower for a delicious and aromatic meal.

17. Balsamic Glazed Pork Tenderloin: Marinate pork tenderloin in a mixture of balsamic vinegar, minced garlic, Dijon mustard, and honey (or a low-carb sweetener). Grill or roast until cooked through, then brush with additional balsamic glaze before serving for a sweet and tangy main dish.

18. Asian Beef Lettuce Wraps: Sauté ground beef with minced garlic, grated ginger, soy sauce, and sesame oil until cooked through. Serve the beef mixture in large lettuce leaves and top with sliced green onions and chopped cilantro for a flavorful and low-carb twist on this classic dish.

19. Cilantro Lime Grilled Chicken: Marinate chicken breasts in a mixture of lime juice, minced garlic, chopped cilantro, and olive oil for at least 30 minutes. Grill until cooked through and serve with a squeeze of fresh lime juice for a bright and zesty main dish.

20. Herb Roasted Turkey Breast: Rub turkey breast with a mixture of chopped fresh herbs like sage, rosemary, and thyme, along with minced garlic and olive oil. Roast until golden and cooked through, then slice and serve with a side of roasted vegetables for a flavorful and satisfying meal.

- Satisfying Snacks for women over 60

Here are some satisfying snacks tailored for women over 60 on the Atkins diet:

1. Cheese and Pepperoni Slices: Enjoy a combination of sliced cheese and pepperoni for a satisfying and protein-rich snack. Opt for full-fat cheese varieties like cheddar, Swiss, or mozzarella, and choose pepperoni slices without added sugars for the best low-carb option.

2. Hard-Boiled Eggs: Hard-boiled eggs are an excellent snack option, providing protein, healthy fats, and essential nutrients. Prepare a batch of hard-boiled eggs ahead of time and enjoy them on their own or sprinkled with a pinch of salt and pepper for extra flavor.

3. Greek Yogurt with Berries: Choose full-fat Greek yogurt and top it with a handful of fresh berries like strawberries, blueberries, or raspberries for a creamy and satisfying snack. Greek yogurt is rich in protein and probiotics, making it a nutritious choice for women over 60.

4. Avocado and Tuna Salad: Mash avocado with canned tuna, diced celery, and a squeeze of lemon juice for a creamy and flavorful snack. Enjoy the avocado and tuna salad on its own or spread it on cucumber slices or celery sticks for added crunch.

5. Celery Sticks with Almond Butter: Spread almond butter on celery sticks for a satisfying and crunchy snack that's rich in healthy fats and protein. Add a sprinkle of cinnamon or a drizzle of honey for extra flavor, if desired.

6. Cheese Crisps: Bake grated cheese in the oven until crispy and golden brown for a crunchy and satisfying snack. Try making cheese crisps with Parmesan, cheddar, or pepper jack cheese for different flavor options.

7. Cucumber and Cream Cheese Roll-Ups: Spread cream cheese on cucumber slices and roll them up for a refreshing and low-carb snack option. Add smoked salmon or deli turkey for extra protein and flavor, if desired.

8. Almonds and Walnuts: Enjoy a handful of almonds or walnuts as a convenient and satisfying snack. Nuts are rich in healthy fats, fiber, and protein, making them an excellent choice for keeping you full and energized between meals.

9. Beef Jerky: Choose beef jerky made with minimal added sugars and preservatives for a portable and protein-packed snack option. Look for beef jerky varieties that are labeled as "sugar-free" or "low-carb" for the best low-carb option.

10. Deviled Eggs: Prepare deviled eggs by filling hard-boiled egg halves with a mixture of mayonnaise, mustard, and seasonings like paprika and black pepper. Deviled eggs are a satisfying and protein-rich snack that's perfect for any time of day.

11. Zucchini Chips: Slice zucchini into thin rounds, toss them with olive oil and seasonings like garlic powder and Italian herbs, then bake until crispy for a crunchy and low-carb snack option.

12. Caprese Skewers: Thread cherry tomatoes, fresh mozzarella balls, and basil leaves onto wooden skewers for a flavorful and portable snack inspired by classic Caprese salad flavors.

13. Cottage Cheese with Cherry Tomatoes: Enjoy cottage cheese topped with halved cherry tomatoes for a creamy and refreshing snack that's rich in protein and calcium.

14. Baked Parmesan Zucchini Fries: Slice zucchini into thin strips, coat them in grated Parmesan cheese and seasonings like garlic powder and Italian herbs, then bake until crispy for a satisfying and low-carb alternative to traditional fries.

15. Smoked Salmon Roll-Ups: Roll smoked salmon slices around cucumber spears or avocado slices for a quick and elegant snack that's rich in omega-3 fatty acids and protein.

- Low-Carb Appetizers for Entertaining

Here are some delicious low-carb appetizers perfect for entertaining that are ideal for women over 60 on the Atkins diet:

1. Stuffed Mushrooms: Fill mushroom caps with a mixture of cream cheese, minced garlic, grated Parmesan cheese, and chopped herbs like parsley or thyme. Bake until the mushrooms are tender and the filling is bubbly for a savory and satisfying appetizer.

2. Cucumber Bites with Smoked Salmon: Slice English cucumber into rounds and top each with a dollop of cream cheese, a piece of smoked salmon, and a sprinkle of chopped chives or dill for a refreshing and elegant appetizer option.

3. Bacon-Wrapped Asparagus Spears: Wrap bundles of asparagus spears with thinly sliced bacon and secure with toothpicks. Bake until the bacon is crispy and the asparagus is tender for a flavorful and easy-to-eat appetizer.

4. Cheese Platter: Arrange a variety of cheeses such as brie, cheddar, and gouda on a platter alongside sliced salami, pepperoni, and prosciutto for a simple yet elegant appetizer option. Add olives, pickles, and nuts for additional flavor and texture.

5. Zucchini Bruschetta: Slice zucchini into rounds and grill or roast until tender. Top each zucchini round with a spoonful of tomato bruschetta topping made with diced tomatoes, minced garlic, olive oil, balsamic vinegar, and chopped basil for a fresh and flavorful appetizer.

6. Cauliflower Hummus with Crudites: Serve cauliflower hummus made with cooked cauliflower, tahini, lemon juice, garlic, and olive oil alongside a variety of raw vegetables like carrots, celery, bell peppers, and cucumber for dipping for a nutritious and low-carb appetizer option.

7. Deviled Eggs with Bacon: Prepare deviled eggs by filling hard-boiled egg halves with a mixture of mayonnaise, mustard, and seasonings like paprika and black pepper. Top each deviled egg with a piece of crispy bacon for an indulgent and flavorful appetizer.

8. Shrimp Cocktail: Serve chilled cooked shrimp with cocktail sauce made with sugar-free ketchup, horseradish, lemon juice, Worcestershire sauce, and hot sauce for a classic and elegant appetizer option that's low in carbs and high in protein.

9. Stuffed Bell Peppers: Halve bell peppers and remove the seeds, then fill each half with a mixture of cream cheese, shredded cheese, cooked sausage or bacon, and chopped green onions. Bake until the peppers are tender and the filling is bubbly for a hearty and flavorful appetizer.

10. Antipasto Skewers: Thread marinated artichoke hearts, cherry tomatoes, mozzarella balls, olives, and salami slices onto wooden skewers for a colorful and flavorful appetizer option that's perfect for entertaining.

11. Eggplant Roll-Ups: Grill or roast slices of eggplant until tender, then roll them up with a mixture of ricotta cheese, minced garlic, chopped basil, and grated Parmesan cheese. Serve the eggplant roll-ups drizzled with marinara sauce for a delicious and low-carb appetizer option.

12. Avocado Stuffed with Crab Salad: Halve avocados and remove the pits, then fill each avocado half with a mixture of lump crab meat, diced celery, mayonnaise, lemon juice, and Old Bay seasoning for a creamy and satisfying appetizer option.

13. Cucumber Sushi Rolls: Slice English cucumber into thin strips using a vegetable peeler, then fill each cucumber strip with a mixture of cooked shrimp, avocado slices, and shredded carrot. Roll up the cucumber strips and secure with toothpicks for a refreshing and low-carb appetizer option.

14. Baked Brie with Almonds: Place a wheel of brie cheese in a baking dish and bake until softened and gooey. Serve the baked brie with sliced almonds and a selection of low-carb crackers or sliced vegetables for dipping for an indulgent and elegant appetizer.

15. Stuffed Jalapenos: Halve jalapeno peppers and remove the seeds, then fill each half with a mixture of cream cheese, shredded cheese, and cooked chorizo or bacon. Bake until the peppers are tender and the filling is bubbly for a spicy and satisfying appetizer option.

- Healthy Nibbles to Keep on Hand

Here are some healthy nibbles to keep on hand for women over 60 on the Atkins diet:

1. Nuts: Keep a variety of nuts such as almonds, walnuts, and pecans on hand for a convenient and nutritious snack option. Nuts are rich in healthy fats, protein, and fiber, making them satisfying and filling.

2. Seeds: Stock up on seeds like pumpkin seeds, sunflower seeds, and chia seeds for a crunchy and nutrient-dense snack option. Seeds are packed with vitamins, minerals, and antioxidants, making them a healthy choice for women over 60.

3. Cheese Crisps: Make homemade cheese crisps by baking grated cheese until crispy and golden brown. Cheese crisps are low in carbs and high in protein, making them a satisfying and flavorful snack option.

4. Vegetable Sticks: Keep a variety of raw vegetable sticks such as carrots, celery, bell peppers, and cucumber on hand for a crunchy and refreshing snack. Pair them with your favorite low-carb dip like guacamole or hummus for added flavor.

5. Hard-Boiled Eggs: Prepare a batch of hard-boiled eggs ahead of time and keep them in the refrigerator for a quick and convenient snack option. Eggs are rich in protein and essential nutrients, making them a nutritious choice for women over 60.

6. Greek Yogurt: Choose full-fat Greek yogurt and keep individual portions on hand for a creamy and satisfying snack option. Greek yogurt is rich in protein and probiotics, making it a nutritious choice for supporting gut health.

7. Canned Tuna or Salmon: Keep canned tuna or salmon on hand for a convenient and protein-rich snack option. Mix it with mayonnaise, mustard, and seasonings for a quick and flavorful tuna or salmon salad.

8. Avocado: Keep ripe avocados on hand for a creamy and nutrient-dense snack option. Enjoy avocado slices on their own or spread them on low-carb crackers or cucumber slices for added texture.

9. Jerky: Choose beef or turkey jerky made with minimal added sugars and preservatives for a portable and protein-packed snack option. Jerky is convenient for on-the-go snacking and can help satisfy hunger between meals.

10. Olives: Keep a jar of olives on hand for a flavorful and satisfying snack option. Olives are low in carbs and rich in healthy fats, making them a nutritious choice for women over 60 on the Atkins diet.

11. Protein Bars: Choose low-carb protein bars made with quality ingredients for a convenient and satisfying snack option. Look for bars that are high in protein and fiber and low in added sugars for the best low-carb option.

12. Cheese Slices: Keep pre-sliced cheese such as cheddar, Swiss, or mozzarella on hand for a quick and satisfying snack option. Cheese is rich in protein and calcium, making it a nutritious choice for women over 60.

13. Edamame: Keep frozen edamame on hand for a convenient and protein-rich snack option. Simply steam or microwave the edamame pods until heated through, then sprinkle with salt and enjoy.

14. Dark Chocolate: Keep a small amount of dark chocolate on hand for a sweet and satisfying snack option. Choose dark chocolate with a high cocoa content and minimal added sugars for the best low-carb option.

15. Low-Carb Crackers: Keep a variety of low-carb crackers on hand for a crunchy and satisfying snack option. Look for crackers made with almond flour, coconut flour, or flaxseed meal for a nutritious choice.

Chapter 8. Desserts and Treats

- Sweet Indulgences for women over 60 on the Atkins Diet

Here are some sweet indulgences suitable for women over 60 on the Atkins Diet:

1. Dark Chocolate: Enjoy a square or two of high-quality dark chocolate with a cocoa content of 70% or higher. Dark chocolate is lower in sugar and higher in antioxidants compared to milk chocolate, making it a satisfying and relatively low-carb treat.

2. Berries with Whipped Cream: Indulge in a serving of fresh berries such as strawberries, raspberries, or blueberries topped with a dollop of unsweetened whipped cream. Berries are naturally lower in carbs compared to other fruits, and when paired with whipped cream, they make for a delicious and satisfying dessert option.

3. Sugar-Free Jello with Whipped Cream: Prepare sugar-free gelatin according to the package instructions and serve it with a dollop of unsweetened whipped cream for a light and refreshing dessert option that's low in carbs and calories.

4. Coconut Macaroons: Make homemade coconut macaroons using shredded coconut, egg whites, and a sugar substitute like erythritol or stevia. These chewy and sweet treats are perfect for satisfying a sweet tooth while keeping carbohydrate intake low.

5. Peanut Butter Fat Bombs: Whip up a batch of peanut butter fat bombs using a mixture of natural peanut butter, coconut oil, and a sugar substitute. These high-fat treats are rich and satisfying, making them perfect for satisfying cravings on the Atkins diet.

6. Cheesecake Mousse: Prepare a creamy and indulgent cheesecake mousse using cream cheese, heavy cream, vanilla extract, and a sugar substitute. Enjoy it on its own or top it with a few berries for added flavor and freshness.

7. Chocolate Avocado Mousse: Blend ripe avocado with unsweetened cocoa powder, a sugar substitute, and a splash of almond milk until smooth and creamy. This rich and chocolatey mousse is packed with healthy fats and fiber, making it a satisfying and nutritious dessert option.

8. Low-Carb Ice Cream: Enjoy a serving of low-carb ice cream made with ingredients like almond milk, heavy cream, and a sugar substitute. Look for commercially available low-carb ice cream options or make your own at home using an ice cream maker.

9. Chia Seed Pudding: Prepare chia seed pudding by soaking chia seeds in almond milk or coconut milk overnight, then sweeten it with a sugar substitute and flavor it with vanilla extract or cocoa powder. Chia seed pudding is creamy, satisfying, and customizable to suit your taste preferences.

10. Almond Flour Cookies: Bake homemade cookies using almond flour, butter, a sugar substitute, and sugar-free chocolate chips or chopped nuts. These cookies are soft, chewy, and satisfying, making them a perfect sweet indulgence for women over 60 on the Atkins diet.

11. Pumpkin Spice Muffins: Bake low-carb pumpkin spice muffins using almond flour, canned pumpkin puree, eggs, a sugar substitute, and warm spices like cinnamon, nutmeg, and cloves. These muffins are moist, flavorful, and perfect for satisfying cravings for fall flavors.

12. Sugar-Free Popsicles: Make homemade sugar-free popsicles using unsweetened fruit juice or herbal tea sweetened with a sugar substitute. Freeze them in popsicle molds for a refreshing and guilt-free dessert option.

13. Lemon Coconut Bars: Prepare lemon coconut bars using almond flour, shredded coconut, eggs, lemon juice, and a sugar substitute. These tangy and sweet bars are reminiscent of lemon bars but with a lower carb count.

14. Chocolate Covered Strawberries: Dip fresh strawberries in melted dark chocolate sweetened with a sugar substitute for a decadent and romantic dessert option that's perfect for special occasions.

15. Almond Butter Cups: Make homemade almond butter cups using dark chocolate, natural almond butter, and a sugar substitute. These rich and creamy treats are reminiscent of peanut butter cups but with a lower carb content.

- Sugar-Free Dessert Options

Here are some sugar-free dessert options suitable for women over 60 on the Atkins diet:

1. Sugar-Free Cheesecake: Prepare a classic cheesecake using cream cheese, eggs, vanilla extract, and a sugar substitute like erythritol or stevia. Bake until set, then chill until firm for a creamy and indulgent dessert option.

2. Sugar-Free Chocolate Pudding: Make homemade chocolate pudding using unsweetened cocoa powder, heavy cream, egg yolks, and a sugar substitute. Cook until thickened, then chill until set for a rich and satisfying dessert option.

3. Sugar-Free Berry Cobbler: Bake a berry cobbler using a mixture of fresh or frozen berries, almond flour, butter, and a sugar substitute. Top with a crumbly almond flour topping and bake until golden brown for a delicious and fruity dessert option.

4. Sugar-Free Lemon Bars: Prepare lemon bars using almond flour, eggs, lemon juice, and a sugar substitute for the crust and filling. Bake until set, then chill until firm for a tangy and refreshing dessert option.

5. Sugar-Free Coconut Macaroons: Make coconut macaroons using shredded coconut, egg whites, vanilla extract, and a sugar substitute like erythritol or stevia. Bake until golden brown and crispy for a chewy and sweet dessert option.

6. Sugar-Free Peanut Butter Cookies: Bake peanut butter cookies using natural peanut butter, almond flour, eggs, vanilla extract, and a sugar substitute. These soft and chewy cookies are perfect for satisfying a sweet tooth without the added sugar.

7. Sugar-Free Chocolate Truffles: Prepare chocolate truffles using unsweetened chocolate, heavy cream, and a sugar substitute like erythritol or stevia. Roll the truffles in cocoa powder or chopped nuts for added flavor and texture.

8. Sugar-Free Coconut Cream Pie: Make a coconut cream pie using coconut milk, eggs, vanilla extract, and a sugar substitute for the filling, and a mixture of almond flour, shredded coconut, butter, and a sugar substitute for the crust. Chill until set for a creamy and indulgent dessert option.

9. Sugar-Free Chocolate Mousse: Whip up a batch of chocolate mousse using heavy cream, unsweetened cocoa powder, vanilla extract, and a sugar substitute. Chill until firm for a rich and decadent dessert option.

10. Sugar-Free Pumpkin Pie: Prepare a pumpkin pie using canned pumpkin puree, eggs, heavy cream, pumpkin pie spice, and a sugar substitute for the filling, and a mixture of almond flour, butter, and a sugar substitute for the crust. Bake until set for a classic and comforting dessert option.

11. Sugar-Free Vanilla Ice Cream: Make homemade vanilla ice cream using heavy cream, egg yolks, vanilla extract, and a sugar substitute like erythritol or stevia. Churn in an ice cream maker until creamy and frozen for a refreshing and satisfying dessert option.

12. Sugar-Free Lemon Cheesecake Bars: Bake lemon cheesecake bars using almond flour, cream cheese, eggs, lemon juice, and a sugar substitute for the crust and filling. Chill until set for a tangy and creamy dessert option.

13. Sugar-Free Chocolate Bark: Melt sugar-free chocolate and spread it onto a baking sheet lined with parchment paper. Sprinkle with chopped nuts, coconut flakes, or dried berries, then chill until set. Break into pieces for a crunchy and indulgent dessert option.

14. Sugar-Free Apple Crisp: Make apple crisp using sliced apples tossed with cinnamon, almond flour, butter, and a sugar substitute for the topping. Bake until bubbly and golden brown for a comforting and satisfying dessert option.

15. Sugar-Free Raspberry Chia Seed Pudding: Prepare chia seed pudding using almond milk, chia seeds, vanilla extract, and a sugar substitute. Layer with fresh raspberries for a nutritious and satisfying dessert option.

   - Simple and Delicious Treats to Satisfy Cravings

Here are some simple and delicious treats to satisfy cravings for women over 60 on the Atkins diet:

1. Cheese Crisps: Bake grated cheese until crispy and golden brown for a crunchy and savory treat that's perfect for satisfying cravings for something salty.

2. Chocolate-Covered Almonds: Dip roasted almonds in melted dark chocolate and let them cool until the chocolate hardens for a satisfying and indulgent treat that's perfect for satisfying cravings for something sweet and crunchy.

3. Cucumber Sandwiches: Slice cucumber into rounds and top each with a small piece of cheese and deli meat for a light and refreshing treat that's perfect for satisfying cravings for something savory and filling.

4. Avocado Chocolate Mousse: Blend ripe avocado with unsweetened cocoa powder, a sugar substitute, and a splash of almond milk until smooth and creamy for a rich and indulgent treat that's perfect for satisfying cravings for something creamy and chocolatey.

5. Berries with Whipped Cream: Enjoy a serving of fresh berries topped with a dollop of unsweetened whipped cream for a simple and satisfying treat that's perfect for satisfying cravings for something sweet and fruity.

6. Greek Yogurt Parfait: Layer full-fat Greek yogurt with fresh berries and a sprinkle of chopped nuts for a creamy and satisfying treat that's perfect for satisfying cravings for something creamy and crunchy.

7. Peanut Butter Celery Sticks: Spread natural peanut butter on celery sticks for a satisfying and crunchy treat that's perfect for satisfying cravings for something savory and filling.

8. Cottage Cheese with Cinnamon: Enjoy a serving of cottage cheese sprinkled with cinnamon for a simple and satisfying treat that's perfect for satisfying cravings for something creamy and lightly sweetened.

9. Hard-Boiled Eggs with Salt: Enjoy a hard-boiled egg sprinkled with salt for a satisfying and protein-rich treat that's perfect for satisfying cravings for something savory and filling.

10. Almond Butter on Apple Slices: Spread natural almond butter on apple slices for a satisfying and crunchy treat that's perfect for satisfying cravings for something sweet and crunchy.

11. Smoked Salmon Roll-Ups: Roll smoked salmon slices around cucumber spears or avocado slices for a satisfying and indulgent treat that's perfect for satisfying cravings for something savory and creamy.

12. Cheese and Pepperoni Roll-Ups: Roll slices of cheese and pepperoni together for a satisfying and savory treat that's perfect for satisfying cravings for something salty and filling.

13. Chocolate Avocado Smoothie: Blend ripe avocado with unsweetened cocoa powder, a sugar substitute, and a splash of almond milk for a creamy and satisfying treat that's perfect for satisfying cravings for something sweet and chocolatey.

14. Almond Flour Pancakes with Berries: Make almond flour pancakes and top them with fresh berries for a satisfying and indulgent treat that's perfect for satisfying cravings for something sweet and comforting.

15. Bacon-Wrapped Asparagus Spears: Wrap bundles of asparagus spears with thinly sliced bacon and bake until crispy for a satisfying and savory treat that's perfect for satisfying cravings for something salty and crunchy.

- Hydrating Drink Options for women over 60

Here are some hydrating drink options suitable for women over 60 on the Atkins diet:

1. Water: Staying hydrated is essential, so drinking plain water throughout the day should be a priority. Aim to drink at least 8 glasses of water per day, or more if you're physically active or live in a hot climate.

2. Herbal Tea: Enjoy a variety of herbal teas such as peppermint, chamomile, or ginger tea. Herbal teas are hydrating and caffeine-free, making them a soothing and refreshing option for staying hydrated throughout the day.

3. Iced Green Tea: Brew green tea and chill it in the refrigerator for a refreshing and hydrating drink option. Green tea is rich in antioxidants and can help support overall health while keeping you hydrated.

4. Infused Water: Add slices of cucumber, lemon, lime, or berries to a pitcher of water for a flavorful and refreshing drink option. Infused water adds natural flavor without any added sugars or calories, making it a healthy and hydrating choice.

5. Coconut Water: Enjoy coconut water as a natural and hydrating drink option. Coconut water is rich in electrolytes like potassium and magnesium, making it a great choice for replenishing hydration levels after exercise or on hot days.

6. Sparkling Water: Enjoy sparkling water with a splash of lemon or lime juice for a refreshing and bubbly drink option. Sparkling water is hydrating and calorie-free, making it a great choice for staying hydrated without any added sugars or artificial sweeteners.

7. Homemade Electrolyte Drink: Make a homemade electrolyte drink using water, lemon juice, a pinch of sea salt, and a small amount of sugar substitute. This homemade electrolyte drink can help replenish electrolytes lost through sweat and support hydration levels.

8. Vegetable Juice: Enjoy vegetable juice made from fresh vegetables like cucumber, celery, kale, and spinach for a hydrating and nutrient-rich drink option. Vegetable juice is low in carbs and calories, making it a healthy choice for women over 60 on the Atkins diet.

9. Bone Broth: Sip on warm bone broth for a hydrating and nourishing drink option. Bone broth is rich in collagen, protein, and minerals, making it a great choice for supporting overall health and hydration.

10. Sugar-Free Iced Tea: Brew unsweetened iced tea and sweeten it with a sugar substitute like stevia or erythritol for a refreshing and hydrating drink option. Add lemon or mint for extra flavor, if desired.

11. Homemade Lemonade: Make homemade lemonade using fresh lemon juice, water, and a sugar substitute. This refreshing drink option is hydrating and low in carbs, making it suitable for women over 60 on the Atkins diet.

12. Flavored Sparkling Water: Enjoy flavored sparkling water with natural flavors like cucumber, watermelon, or mint for a refreshing and hydrating drink option. Flavored sparkling water adds variety without any added sugars or calories.

13. Hibiscus Tea: Brew hibiscus tea and enjoy it hot or cold for a hydrating and antioxidant-rich drink option. Hibiscus tea is naturally caffeine-free and can help support heart health and hydration.

14. Lemon Ginger Detox Water: Infuse water with slices of lemon and ginger for a hydrating and detoxifying drink option. Lemon and ginger add natural flavor and can help support digestion and hydration.

15. Homemade Electrolyte Popsicles: Make homemade electrolyte popsicles using coconut water, fruit juice, and a pinch of sea salt for a hydrating and refreshing treat option. These homemade popsicles are perfect for staying hydrated on hot days.

- Low-Carb Beverage Choices

Here are some low-carb beverage choices for women over 60 on the Atkins diet:

1. Unsweetened Almond Milk: Enjoy unsweetened almond milk as a low-carb alternative to dairy milk. It's creamy and flavorful, with fewer carbs than regular milk, making it suitable for those following a low-carb diet.

2. Unsweetened Coconut Milk: Opt for unsweetened coconut milk as another dairy-free and low-carb beverage option. It has a rich and creamy texture, making it a great addition to smoothies or enjoyed on its own.

3. Bulletproof Coffee: Blend brewed coffee with grass-fed butter and coconut oil or MCT oil for a creamy and satisfying low-carb beverage option. Bulletproof coffee provides sustained energy and can be enjoyed as a breakfast replacement for those following intermittent fasting or keto diets.

4. Sugar-Free Flavored Syrups: Add sugar-free flavored syrups to coffee or tea for a sweet and flavorful low-carb beverage option. Look for syrups sweetened with erythritol or stevia instead of sugar for a healthier alternative.

5. Unsweetened Iced Tea: Brew unsweetened tea and chill it in the refrigerator for a refreshing and hydrating low-carb beverage option. Enjoy it plain or with a splash of lemon or lime juice for added flavor.

6. Sugar-Free Energy Drinks: Choose sugar-free energy drinks sweetened with artificial sweeteners like sucralose or aspartame for a low-carb and energizing beverage option. However, be mindful of caffeine content and consume in moderation.

7. Kombucha: Select low-carb kombucha varieties for a tangy and probiotic-rich beverage option. Look for kombucha brands with minimal added sugars and carbohydrates to keep carb intake low.

8. Unsweetened Sparkling Water: Enjoy plain sparkling water or flavored sparkling water without added sugars for a bubbly and refreshing low-carb beverage option. Add a squeeze of lemon or lime for extra flavor, if desired.

9. Sugar-Free Protein Shakes: Opt for sugar-free protein shakes made with water or unsweetened almond milk for a convenient and low-carb beverage option. Look for protein powders with minimal added sugars and carbohydrates for the best low-carb option.

10. Low-Carb Smoothies: Blend together unsweetened almond milk, spinach or kale, protein powder, and a small portion of low-carb fruits like berries for a nutritious and filling low-carb beverage option. Customize the ingredients based on your preferences and dietary needs.

11. Bone Broth: Sip on warm bone broth for a nourishing and low-carb beverage option. Bone broth is rich in collagen, protein, and minerals, making it a great choice for supporting overall health and hydration.

12. Unsweetened Herbal Infusions: Brew herbal infusions like peppermint, chamomile, or hibiscus tea for a soothing and low-carb beverage option. Herbal infusions are caffeine-free and can be enjoyed hot or cold.

13. Vinegar Drinks: Mix apple cider vinegar with water and a sugar substitute for a tart and refreshing low-carb beverage option. Apple cider vinegar may offer various health benefits, including improved digestion and blood sugar control.

14. Low-Carb Vegetable Juice: Blend together low-carb vegetables like cucumber, celery, and spinach with water or unsweetened almond milk for a nutrient-rich and low-carb beverage option. Add a splash of lemon or lime juice for extra flavor.

15. Low-Carb Cocktails: Enjoy low-carb cocktails made with spirits like vodka, gin, or tequila mixed with soda water and a splash of lime or lemon juice for a refreshing and low-carb beverage option. Avoid sugary mixers and syrups to keep carb intake low.

 - Mocktail and Cocktail Recipes
Here are some mocktail and cocktail recipes suitable for women over 60 on the Atkins diet:

Mocktail Recipes:

1. Virgin Mojito:
  - Ingredients: Fresh mint leaves, lime wedges, soda water, sugar substitute, ice.
  - Instructions: Muddle mint leaves and lime wedges in a glass. Add ice, soda water, and a sugar substitute to taste. Stir well and garnish with a mint sprig.

2. Cucumber Cooler:
  - Ingredients: Cucumber slices, lime juice, soda water, sugar substitute, ice.
  - Instructions: Blend cucumber slices and lime juice until smooth. Strain the mixture into a glass filled with ice. Top with soda water and a sugar substitute to taste. Stir gently and garnish with a cucumber slice.

3. Berry Sparkler:
  - Ingredients: Mixed berries (such as strawberries, raspberries, and blueberries), sparkling water, lemon juice, sugar substitute, ice.
  - Instructions: Muddle mixed berries in a glass. Add ice, sparkling water, lemon juice, and a sugar substitute to taste. Stir gently and garnish with a lemon slice.

4. Pineapple Mint Spritzer:

- Ingredients: Pineapple juice (unsweetened), fresh mint leaves, soda water, lime juice, sugar substitute, ice.

- Instructions: In a glass, muddle fresh mint leaves with lime juice. Add ice, pineapple juice, soda water, and a sugar substitute to taste. Stir well and garnish with a mint sprig.

5. Watermelon Basil Cooler:

- Ingredients: Watermelon chunks, fresh basil leaves, lime juice, soda water, sugar substitute, ice.

- Instructions: Blend watermelon chunks and basil leaves until smooth. Strain the mixture into a glass filled with ice. Add lime juice, soda water, and a sugar substitute to taste. Stir gently and garnish with a basil leaf.

Cocktail Recipes:

1. Keto Margarita:

- Ingredients: Tequila, fresh lime juice, orange extract, sugar substitute, ice, salt (for rimming, optional).

- Instructions: In a shaker, combine tequila, lime juice, orange extract, and a sugar substitute to taste. Shake well with ice. Strain into a salt-rimmed glass filled with ice. Garnish with a lime wedge.

2. Low-Carb Mojito:

- Ingredients: White rum, fresh mint leaves, lime wedges, soda water, sugar substitute, ice.

- Instructions: Muddle mint leaves and lime wedges in a glass. Add rum, a sugar substitute to taste, and ice. Top with soda water and stir gently. Garnish with a mint sprig.

3. Skinny Cosmopolitan:

- Ingredients: Vodka, unsweetened cranberry juice, fresh lime juice, orange extract, sugar substitute, ice.

- Instructions: In a shaker, combine vodka, cranberry juice, lime juice, orange extract, and a sugar substitute to taste. Shake well with ice. Strain into a martini glass and garnish with a lime twist.

4. Low-Carb Mojito Royale:

   - Ingredients: White rum, fresh mint leaves, lime wedges, sparkling water, sugar-free ginger ale, sugar substitute, ice.

   - Instructions: Muddle mint leaves and lime wedges in a glass. Add rum, a sugar substitute to taste, and ice. Top with equal parts sparkling water and sugar-free ginger ale. Stir gently and garnish with a mint sprig.

5. Gin and Tonic Twist:

   - Ingredients: Gin, sugar-free tonic water, fresh lime juice, cucumber slices, sugar substitute, ice.

   - Instructions: In a glass, combine gin, tonic water, lime juice, cucumber slices, and a sugar substitute to taste. Stir well and add ice. Garnish with a cucumber slice and a lime wedge.

Chapter 10. Special Considerations for Older women

- Addressing Common Concerns

Here are some common concerns for women over 60 on the Atkins diet and how to address them:

1. Low Energy Levels: Some women may experience low energy levels when starting the Atkins diet, especially during the initial phase of carbohydrate restriction. To address this concern, focus on consuming adequate protein and healthy fats to provide sustained energy throughout the day. Additionally, staying hydrated and incorporating low-carb vegetables can help maintain energy levels and prevent fatigue.

2. Digestive Issues: Transitioning to a low-carb diet like Atkins may cause digestive issues such as constipation or bloating for some women. To alleviate these symptoms, ensure you're consuming enough fiber from non-starchy vegetables, nuts, seeds, and low-carb fruits like berries. Drinking plenty of water and incorporating probiotic-rich foods like yogurt or fermented vegetables can also support digestive health.

3. Muscle Loss: Concerns about muscle loss may arise, especially if protein intake is insufficient or if exercise levels decrease while following the Atkins diet. To preserve muscle mass, prioritize protein-rich foods such as meat, poultry, fish, eggs, and tofu. Engage in regular strength training exercises to maintain muscle mass and promote overall strength and mobility.

4. Bone Health: Some women may worry about the impact of a low-carb diet on bone health, particularly if dairy intake is limited. To support bone health, include calcium-rich foods such as dairy products, leafy green vegetables, tofu, and almonds in your diet. Additionally, ensure adequate vitamin D intake through sun exposure or supplementation to enhance calcium absorption.

5. Dehydration: The initial phase of the Atkins diet may lead to increased water loss and dehydration, especially if carbohydrate intake is significantly reduced. To prevent dehydration, drink plenty of water throughout the day and consider consuming hydrating foods like

cucumbers, tomatoes, and watermelon. Limiting caffeine and alcohol intake can also help maintain hydration levels.

6. Social Challenges: Following a low-carb diet like Atkins may pose challenges in social situations, such as dining out or attending gatherings where carb-heavy foods are served. To navigate social situations, plan ahead by researching restaurant menus for low-carb options or offering to bring a dish that fits your dietary preferences. Communicate your dietary needs to friends and family members to ensure they understand and can accommodate your choices.

7. Micronutrient Deficiencies: Restricting certain food groups on the Atkins diet may increase the risk of micronutrient deficiencies, particularly in nutrients like vitamins C, E, and K, as well as magnesium and potassium. To address this concern, focus on consuming a variety of nutrient-dense foods, including low-carb vegetables, fruits, nuts, seeds, and lean proteins.

8. Long-Term Sustainability: Women over 60 may be concerned about the long-term sustainability of the Atkins diet and whether they can maintain their desired weight loss and health benefits over time. To ensure long-term success, focus on adopting a balanced and varied eating pattern that incorporates whole, minimally processed foods. Gradually reintroduce carbohydrates from nutrient-dense sources like fruits, vegetables, and whole grains while monitoring portion sizes and staying mindful of carb intake.

 - Adjusting the Atkins Diet for Older women Health Needs
Adjusting the Atkins diet for the health needs of older women involves considerations such as metabolism changes, nutrient requirements, bone health, and overall well-being. Here are some key adjustments to make:

1. Focus on Protein: Older women may need more protein to support muscle mass maintenance and repair. Including lean protein sources such as poultry, fish, eggs, tofu, and legumes in each meal can help meet protein needs and support overall health.

2. Emphasize Healthy Fats: While the Atkins diet encourages the consumption of healthy fats, it's essential to prioritize monounsaturated and polyunsaturated fats over saturated fats. Incorporating sources like olive oil, avocado, nuts, seeds, and fatty fish can provide essential fatty acids and support heart health.

3. Increase Fiber Intake: Older women may experience digestive issues like constipation, so it's crucial to include plenty of fiber-rich foods in the diet. Non-starchy vegetables, nuts, seeds, and low-carb fruits like berries are excellent sources of fiber that can support digestive health and regularity.

4. Monitor Carbohydrate Intake: Adjusting carbohydrate intake based on individual needs and preferences is essential. While some older women may thrive on a low-carb approach, others may benefit from a moderate-carb or cyclical ketogenic approach. Experiment with carb levels and pay attention to how your body responds to find the right balance.

5. Prioritize Bone Health: Older women are at increased risk of osteoporosis, so it's essential to prioritize bone health. Include calcium-rich foods like dairy products, leafy green vegetables, and fortified plant-based milk alternatives in the diet. Additionally, ensure adequate vitamin D intake through sun exposure, supplementation, or fortified foods to support calcium absorption.

6. Stay Hydrated: Dehydration can be more common in older adults, so it's crucial to stay hydrated throughout the day. Aim to drink plenty of water and incorporate hydrating foods like cucumbers, tomatoes, and watermelon into meals and snacks.

7. Consider Nutrient Supplementation: Older women may have higher nutrient requirements or difficulty absorbing certain nutrients, so supplementation may be necessary. Discuss with a healthcare professional to determine if supplements such as calcium, vitamin D, vitamin B12, or omega-3 fatty acids are needed based on individual health needs and dietary intake.

8. Mindful Eating: Pay attention to hunger and satiety cues, and practice mindful eating to avoid overeating and promote enjoyment of meals. Eating slowly, savoring flavors, and focusing on nutrient-dense foods can support overall well-being and satisfaction with the diet.

9. Regular Physical Activity: Incorporating regular physical activity into your routine can support weight management, muscle strength, bone density, and overall health. Engage in activities like walking, strength training, yoga, or swimming to promote physical and mental well-being.

10. Listen to Your Body: Lastly, listen to your body and adjust the diet as needed based on how you feel. If certain foods or eating patterns don't agree with you, don't hesitate to make changes to optimize your health and well-being.

- Staying Motivated

Staying motivated on the Atkins diet, or any dietary regimen, can be challenging at times, but there are several strategies you can use to maintain your enthusiasm and commitment. Here are some tips specifically tailored for women over 60 on the Atkins diet:

1. Set Realistic Goals: Establish achievable and realistic goals that are specific, measurable, and time-bound. Break down larger goals into smaller milestones to track progress and celebrate achievements along the way.

2. Focus on Non-Scale Victories: Instead of solely focusing on the number on the scale, celebrate non-scale victories such as increased energy levels, improved mood, better sleep, or looser-fitting clothes. These positive changes can be powerful motivators and indicators of progress.

3. Find Support: Seek support from friends, family members, or online communities who understand and support your dietary goals. Surrounding yourself with like-minded individuals can provide encouragement, accountability, and motivation during challenging times.

4. Experiment with Recipes: Keep your meals exciting and enjoyable by experimenting with new recipes and flavors that fit within the Atkins guidelines.

5. Keep Track of Progress: Keep a food journal or use a mobile app to track your food intake, physical activity, and progress towards your goals. Monitoring your daily habits and behaviors can help identify areas for improvement and reinforce positive changes over time.

6. Reward Yourself: Set up a reward system to celebrate reaching milestones or sticking to your dietary plan. Treat yourself to non-food rewards such as a relaxing spa day, a new book, or a fun outing with friends as a way to acknowledge your hard work and dedication.

7. Practice Self-Compassion: Be kind to yourself and practice self-compassion, especially during setbacks or moments of temptation. Remember that nobody is perfect, and it's okay to slip up

occasionally. Focus on progress, not perfection, and use setbacks as learning opportunities to make adjustments and move forward.

8. Visualize Success: Visualize yourself achieving your health and wellness goals, whether it's fitting into a favorite outfit, participating in an activity you love, or enjoying improved health outcomes. Creating a mental image of success can help reinforce your motivation and keep you focused on your long-term objectives.

9. Practice Mindfulness: Incorporate mindfulness techniques such as meditation, deep breathing exercises, or mindful eating practices into your daily routine. Mindfulness can help reduce stress, improve self-awareness, and enhance your ability to make conscious and intentional decisions about food and lifestyle choices.

- Tracking Progress

Tracking your progress on the Atkins diet is an excellent way to stay motivated and monitor your journey towards achieving your health and wellness goals. Here are some effective methods for tracking your progress as a woman over 60 on the Atkins diet:

1. Keep a Food Journal: Record everything you eat and drink throughout the day, including portion sizes and carbohydrate counts. A food journal can help you identify patterns, track your carb intake, and make adjustments as needed to stay on track with the Atkins diet.

2. Use a Mobile App: Utilize a mobile app designed for tracking nutrition and fitness, such as MyFitnessPal, Lose It!, or Atkins Carb Counter. These apps allow you to log your meals, track your daily macronutrient intake (carbs, protein, and fat), monitor your progress, and set personalized goals.

3. Track Weight Loss: Weigh yourself regularly, ideally once a week, and record your progress over time. Keep track of your weight loss journey using a spreadsheet, a weight tracking app, or a journal to visualize your progress and stay motivated.

4. Measure Body Measurements: Take measurements of key areas of your body, such as your waist, hips, thighs, and arms, using a measuring tape. Record these measurements regularly and track changes over time to monitor changes in body composition and inches lost.

5. Monitor Energy Levels and Well-Being: Pay attention to how you feel on a daily basis, including your energy levels, mood, sleep quality, and overall well-being. Keep a journal to track any changes or improvements in these areas as you progress on the Atkins diet.

6. Keep a Fitness Log: If you're incorporating exercise into your routine, keep a log of your workouts, including the type of activity, duration, and intensity. Tracking your physical activity can help you stay accountable and monitor improvements in strength, endurance, and fitness level over time.

7. Take Progress Photos: Take before photos at the start of your Atkins journey and periodic progress photos along the way. Comparing photos side by side can provide visual evidence of your transformation and serve as a powerful reminder of how far you've come.

8. Monitor Blood Sugar Levels: If you have diabetes or are at risk of developing diabetes, monitor your blood sugar levels regularly to track changes in response to your dietary changes. Consult with a healthcare professional for guidance on monitoring blood sugar levels and interpreting the results.

9. Keep a Daily Log: Maintain a daily log or journal where you can record your meals, snacks, water intake, physical activity, and any observations or reflections about your progress on the Atkins diet. Reviewing your daily log can help you identify areas for improvement and celebrate successes.

10. Set Specific Goals: Set specific and measurable goals related to your health, weight loss, fitness, or overall well-being. Break down larger goals into smaller, actionable steps, and track your progress towards achieving them over time.

- Long-Term Strategies for Health and Wellness

As a woman over 60 following the Atkins diet, adopting long-term strategies for health and wellness is crucial for maintaining overall well-being and achieving sustainable results. Here are some effective long-term strategies to consider:

1. Focus on Whole Foods: Emphasize whole, minimally processed foods that are nutrient-dense and rich in vitamins, minerals, and antioxidants. Incorporate a variety of colorful fruits and vegetables, lean proteins, healthy fats, and high-fiber carbohydrates into your diet to ensure you're meeting your nutritional needs and supporting long-term health.

2. Maintain a Balanced Diet: Strive for balance and moderation in your dietary choices, even while following the Atkins diet. Aim to include a variety of food groups in your meals to ensure you're getting a wide range of nutrients and avoiding nutrient deficiencies. Listen to your body's hunger and fullness cues and eat mindfully to prevent overeating.

3. Stay Active: Incorporate regular physical activity into your routine to support overall health, mobility, and quality of life. Engage in a variety of activities that you enjoy, including cardiovascular exercise, strength training, flexibility exercises, and balance exercises. Aim for at least 150 minutes of moderate-intensity aerobic activity or 75 minutes of vigorous-intensity aerobic activity per week, as recommended by the American Heart Association.

4. Prioritize Bone Health: As a woman over 60, maintaining strong and healthy bones is essential for preventing osteoporosis and reducing the risk of fractures. Ensure you're getting an adequate intake of calcium and vitamin D through dietary sources or supplements, engage in weight-bearing exercises like walking or strength training, and avoid smoking and excessive alcohol consumption, which can weaken bones.

5. Manage Stress: Practice stress management techniques such as meditation, deep breathing exercises, yoga, tai chi, or mindfulness to reduce stress levels and promote relaxation. Chronic stress can have negative effects on both physical and mental health, so prioritizing stress reduction is essential for overall well-being.

6. Get Quality Sleep: Aim for 7-9 hours of quality sleep per night to support optimal health and wellness. Practice good sleep hygiene habits such as establishing a regular sleep schedule, creating a relaxing bedtime routine, minimizing screen time before bed, and creating a comfortable sleep environment to improve sleep quality and duration.

7. Stay Hydrated: Drink plenty of water throughout the day to stay hydrated and support overall health. Aim for at least 8 glasses of water per day, or more if you're physically active or live in a hot climate. Avoid excessive consumption of sugary beverages and alcohol, which can contribute to dehydration and other health issues.

8. Regular Health Check-Ups: Schedule regular health check-ups with your healthcare provider to monitor your health, address any concerns or changes in your health status, and receive preventive screenings and vaccinations as recommended for your age and medical history. Be proactive about managing any chronic conditions or risk factors to optimize your long-term health and wellness.

9. Practice Self-Care: Prioritize self-care activities that promote relaxation, enjoyment, and overall well-being. Take time for activities you love, such as hobbies, reading, spending time with loved ones, or engaging in creative pursuits. Nurturing your mental and emotional health is just as important as caring for your physical health.

10. Stay Educated: Stay informed about the latest research, guidelines, and recommendations related to nutrition, health, and wellness. Continuously educate yourself about topics relevant to aging gracefully and maintaining optimal health as a woman over 60.

<u>Chapter 12. Conclusion</u>

- Final Thoughts and Encouragement

As you embark on your journey with the Atkins diet as a woman over 60, it's essential to remember that you're taking positive steps towards improving your health, well-being, and quality of life. Here are some final thoughts and words of encouragement to support you along the way:

1. Celebrate Your Progress: Celebrate every milestone, no matter how small. Whether it's losing a few pounds, feeling more energetic, or making healthier food choices, each step forward is a victory worth acknowledging and celebrating. Be proud of your accomplishments and the efforts you're making to prioritize your health.

2. Be Patient and Persistent: Remember that change takes time, and progress may not always happen as quickly as you'd like. Stay patient and persistent in your efforts, even when faced with challenges or setbacks. Focus on making gradual, sustainable changes that you can maintain over the long term.

3. Listen to Your Body: Pay attention to how your body feels and responds to the Atkins diet. Tune in to hunger and fullness cues, and adjust your dietary choices accordingly. Trust your instincts and prioritize self-care, listening to what your body needs to thrive.

4. Embrace Flexibility: While the Atkins diet provides a framework for healthy eating, it's essential to be flexible and adaptable to your individual needs and preferences. Don't be afraid to experiment with different foods, meal plans, and approaches to find what works best for you. Remember that there's no one-size-fits-all approach to nutrition, and what works for one person may not work for another.

5. Seek Support and Connection: Surround yourself with supportive friends, family members, or online communities who understand and encourage your journey with the Atkins diet. Share your successes, challenges, and experiences with others who can offer guidance, motivation, and empathy along the way.

6. Practice Self-Compassion: Be kind to yourself and practice self-compassion throughout your journey. Accept that perfection is not attainable, and it's okay to make mistakes or slip-ups along the way. Treat yourself with the same kindness and understanding that you would offer to a friend facing similar challenges.

7. Focus on Non-Scale Victories: Shift your focus away from the number on the scale and instead celebrate the non-scale victories that indicate progress and success. Whether it's improved energy levels, better sleep, increased mobility, or a positive mindset, these achievements are just as significant, if not more so, than changes in weight.

8. Stay Inspired and Informed: Stay inspired and motivated by seeking out success stories, testimonials, and resources that resonate with you. Stay informed about the latest research, tips, and strategies related to the Atkins diet and healthy living. Keep learning, growing, and evolving on your journey towards optimal health and wellness.

9. Trust the Process: Trust in yourself and the process of transformation that you're undergoing. Believe in your ability to make positive changes and overcome obstacles along the way. Stay committed to your goals, and remember that every step forward, no matter how small, is progress towards a healthier, happier you.

10. You're Worth It: Finally, remember that your health and well-being are worth investing in. You deserve to feel your best and live life to the fullest, regardless of age or stage in life. Keep prioritizing your health, nurturing your body and mind, and embracing the journey with optimism, resilience, and grace.

As you continue on your journey with the Atkins diet, may you find strength, inspiration, and joy in the process of nourishing your body, mind, and spirit. You have the power to create positive change and transform your life in ways you never imagined. Believe in yourself, stay committed to your goals, and know that you're capable of achieving anything you set your mind to.

-Carb Counting Charts

Creating a carb counting chart for the Atkins diet involves categorizing foods based on their carbohydrate content and providing guidelines for portion sizes.

Here is a simplified example of a carb counting chart for the Atkins diet:

Food Category	Examples	Carb Content (grams)
Vegetables	Leafy greens (spinach, kale, lettuce), cruciferous vegetables (broccoli, cauliflower, Brussels sprouts), peppers, cucumbers, zucchini, mushrooms	0-5 grams per serving
Berries	Strawberries, raspberries, blackberries	5-10 grams per 1/2 cup
Other fruits	Avocado, tomatoes, lemon, lime	5-10 grams per serving
Nuts and seeds	Almonds, walnuts, pecans, chia seeds, flaxseeds	1-5 grams per serving
Diary products	Full-fat cheese, cream, Greek yogurt (unsweetened)	0-10 grams per serving
Protein sources	Beef, poultry, fish, seafood, tofu, tempeh	0 grams per serving
Fats and oils	Olive oil, coconut oil, avocado oil, butter, ghee	0 grams per serving

Note: Portion sizes and carb contents may vary depending on the specific food and brand. Always check nutrition labels to determine accurate carb counts.

-Glossary of terms

Here's a glossary of terms relevant to the Atkins diet for women over 60:

1. Atkins Diet: A low-carbohydrate diet developed by Dr. Robert Atkins that emphasizes high protein and fat intake while limiting carbohydrates to induce weight loss and improve overall health.

2. Net Carbs: The total carbohydrate content of a food minus the fiber and sugar alcohols, which are not fully absorbed by the body and do not impact blood sugar levels as much as other carbohydrates.

3. Induction Phase: The initial phase of the Atkins diet, typically lasting two weeks, during which carbohydrate intake is restricted to 20-25 grams per day to transition the body into ketosis and kickstart weight loss.

4. Ketosis: A metabolic state in which the body switches from using glucose as its primary fuel source to using ketones, which are produced from fat stores. Ketosis is induced by carbohydrate restriction and is a key component of the Atkins diet.

5. Fat Adaptation: The process by which the body becomes more efficient at burning fat for fuel, typically occurring after several weeks of following a low-carb, high-fat diet like Atkins.

6. OWL (Ongoing Weight Loss): The second phase of the Atkins diet, during which carbohydrate intake is gradually increased to find an individual's tolerance level for weight loss while still maintaining ketosis.

7. Pre-Maintenance: The phase of the Atkins diet in which carbohydrate intake is further increased to prepare for transitioning to the maintenance phase while still promoting gradual weight loss.

8. Maintenance Phase: The final phase of the Atkins diet, during which carbohydrate intake is adjusted to maintain weight loss and support long-term health and wellness.

9. Foundation Vegetables: Low-carb vegetables that can be consumed freely throughout all phases of the Atkins diet, including leafy greens, cruciferous vegetables, peppers, cucumbers, and tomatoes.

10. Low-Carb Flu: Temporary symptoms such as fatigue, headache, dizziness, and irritability that some individuals experience during the initial phase of the Atkins diet as the body adjusts to ketosis and shifts its primary fuel source from carbohydrates to fat.

11. Carb Creep: The unintentional increase in carbohydrate intake over time, often due to consuming small amounts of high-carb foods or beverages that can add up and hinder weight loss or ketosis.

12. Sugar Alcohols: Low-calorie sweeteners found in some sugar-free and low-carb foods and beverages, such as erythritol, xylitol, and maltitol, which provide sweetness without significantly impacting blood sugar levels.

13. Hydration: The importance of drinking plenty of water on the Atkins diet to stay hydrated and support overall health, especially during the initial phase when water loss may increase due to carbohydrate restriction.

14. Meal Planning: The process of preparing meals and snacks in advance to ensure they align with the Atkins diet guidelines and support your health and weight loss goals.

15. Carb Counting: Keeping track of the total carbohydrate content of foods and beverages consumed throughout the day to stay within the recommended carb allowance for each phase of the Atkins diet.

www.ingramcontent.com/pod-product-compliance
Lightning Source LLC
Chambersburg PA
CBHW081223260726
48653CB00010BB/3779